Soft tissue filler complications: prevention and management

Edited by
Jani van Loghem, MD PhD
Philippe Snozzi, MD

Text editor
Aarent Brand Kanters, MD

UMA academy

CRC Press
Taylor & Francis Group
Boca Raton London New York

CRC Press is an imprint of the
Taylor & Francis Group, an **informa** business

Know what can go wrong.
Know what can go right.
Know why something works, and when it won't.
Know the difference between good and great.
Know what a patient wants, and what they need.
Know when to push on. Know when to stop.
Know why you're being cautious, or brave.
Know what you don't know.
Know more than the products in your dispensary.
Know more than the treatments you offer,
or the tools you use to deliver them.
Know how to express who your patient wants to be.

knowledge is beautiful

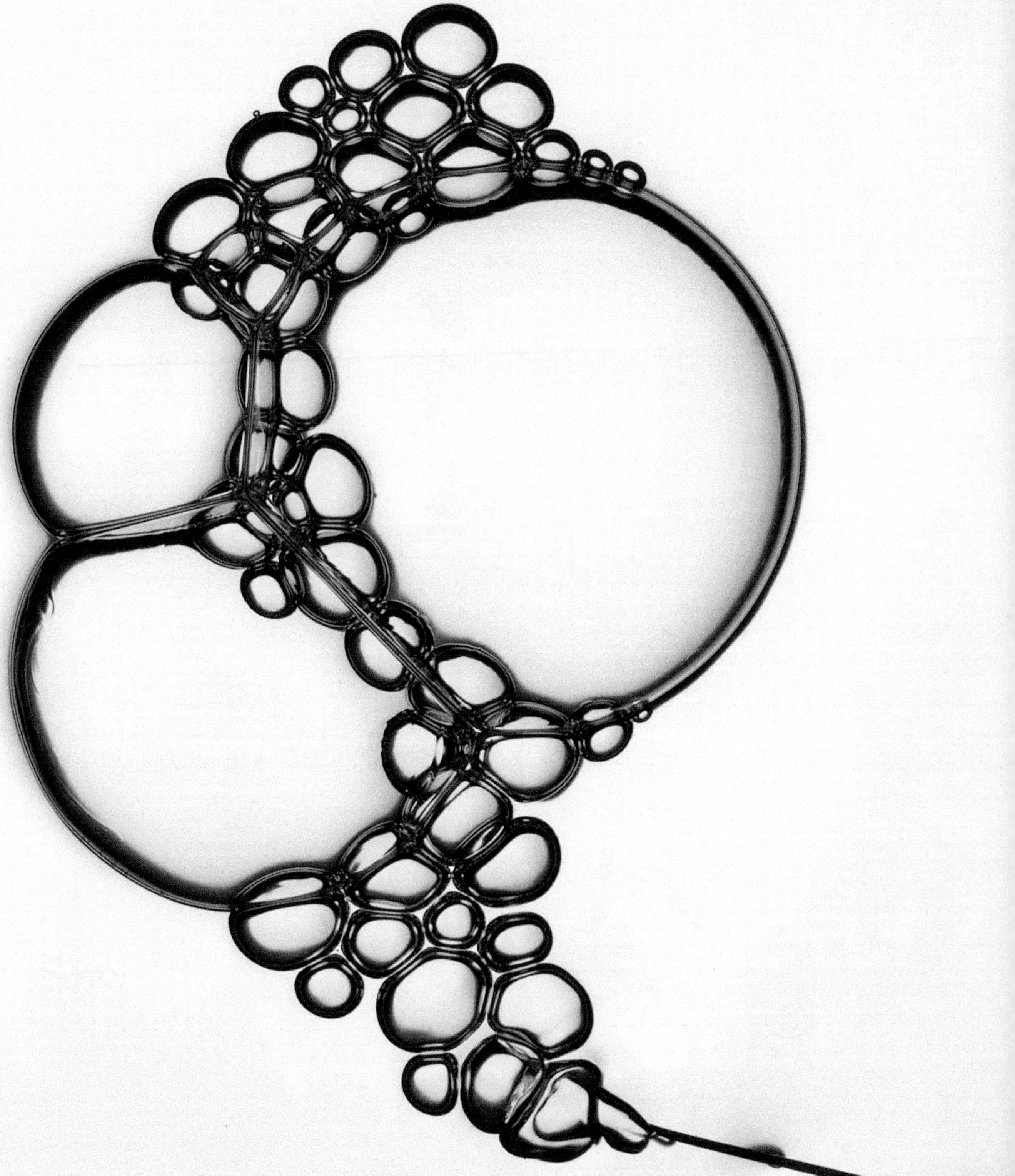

Cover design by UMA
Text design by Rosa Koolhoven and Eszter Takács/Eszter Design
Photography by Bart Oomes
Videos by Casper van der Linden

This edition published 2023
by CRC Press
6000 Broken Sound Parkway NW, Suite 300, Boca Raton, FL 33487-2742

and by CRC Press
4 Park Square, Milton Park, Abingdon, Oxon, OX14 4RN

CRC Press is an imprint of Taylor & Francis Group, LLC

ISBN: 978-1-032-44046-0 (hbk)
ISBN: 978-1-032-44049-1 (pbk)
ISBN: 978-1-003-37015-4 (ebk)

DOI: 10.1201/9781003370154

Typeset in Optima
by KnowledgeWorks Global Ltd.

let's talk about complications

Prevention and Management

table of contents

Introduction by founder 08

01 avoiding and minimalizing complications 11

Introduction 12
1.1 Patient history 14
1.2 Product choice 16
1.3 Anatomy 17
1.4 Injection technique 20
1.5 Needle vs. cannula 22
1.6 Aspiration 22

02 HA, CaHA and PLLA complication management 27

Introduction 28
2.1 Skin discoloration 30
2.2 Edema 35
2.3 Infection 38
2.4 Nodules 41
2.5 Prevention and management of vascular complications 46
2.6 Poly-L-lactic acid (PLLA) complications 58

03 non-resorbable filler complication management 65

Introduction 66
3.1 Granulomas 68
3.2 Non-resorbable filler 73

04 ultrasound imaging in filler complications 79

Introduction 80
4.1 Ultrasound imaging in filler complications 82

05 appendix 89

Introduction 90
5.1 UMA filler first aid kit 92
5.2 Hyaluronidase 93
5.3 Post-treatment scarring 94
5.4 Basic principles for the use of laser therapy in complication management 97
5.5 The future is here – special contributions 100

References 102
About the co-authors and editors 111
Index 118

introduction

Complications after injection of soft tissue fillers (STF) can have a major impact on the quality of life of the patient. It is therefore essential that injectors are up to date with the preventive measures and management of complications due to STF. Different complications can present with similar symptoms, for example, type IV delayed immune reaction versus low-grade infection associated with biofilm. Each requires different treatments, that is, immunosuppression versus antibiotics, although both may have the same medical consequences, that is, granulomatous and fibrotic processes caused by chronic immune stimulation. Similarly, an intravascular event can look like a bruise, but these different complications require very different treatment approaches.

Currently, the most serious complications are technique related vascular embolization resulting in necrosis and/or blindness. As practitioners have moved beyond standard filling of superficial wrinkles and now also inject more risky areas (e.g., nose, forehead, temples, brows, glabella, superior orbital and the infraorbital areas), more serious adverse events (AEs) are being reported in the past years. Besides technique related complications, some products have been associated with delayed inflammatory reactions. This may have to do with the demand for longer lasting, stable results, resulting in innovations in cross-linking of hyaluronic acid (HA) products. Crosslinking changes the three-dimensional structure/shape of injectable HA and it may become more different from human HA than less crosslinked HA, resulting in an increased chance of foreign body reactions. Bacteria may also contribute to this reaction and the patient's immune status has an impact as well, so these kind of complications have all three factors included in the pathogenesis of late inflammatory reactions.

Over the past decades, a steady growth has been recorded of the use of STF and millions of STF treatments are performed every year.[1] With that, the number of complications is also rising. In recent years, the providers of STFs have grown in numbers and have grown beyond the realm of the medical doctor. Dentists, physician assistants, nurse practitioners and even non-medical workers, such as beauticians have begun to inject STFs into their clients. As reputable pharmaceutical companies do not provide their products to non-medical practitioners, there is an increasing demand for black market products, parallel import and copycat products of which the quality cannot be assured. For physicians with a medical license, it is easy to access the market of soft tissue fillers. In many countries, all that is required is to follow a workshop organized by a pharmaceutical company and after that, the physician can buy products and start his/her own clinic. Beginning clinics with beginner providers usually have low prices to compete on the market, which leads to limited time per patient. These ingredients together may form a recipe for STF complications.

In The Netherlands, aesthetic medicine is registered as a medical specialty and a 2-year fulltime training program is obligatory. After successful completion, the physician is awarded with a protected title (in the Netherlands it's Aesthetic Physician, KNMG). This title differentiates well-trained aesthetic physicians from other providers and serves as quality assurance for patients.

Registration of complications is generally mandatory with most professional societies for aesthetic physicians. The purpose of truthful registration of complications is to get a detailed understanding on the incidence of each complication, but it also gives the opportunity to learn from each other so similar complications can be avoided in the future. Diagnoses are usually based on the clinical presentation, with further investigations (e.g., biopsy, bacteriology) being difficult or nonspecific (e.g., general laboratory tests). Most recommendations for management of complications are based on expert opinions, with little data available from controlled studies. This is because clinical trials are difficult to conduct since patients are usually treated in private practices, and patients generally demand fast treatment and recovery, without the burden associated with a clinical study.

The purpose of this book is to provide the aesthetic practitioner with theoretical backgrounds regarding the most common and serious complications arising from HA, calcium hydroxylapatite (CaHA) filler treatments as well as PLLA and non-resorbable filler treatments. We hope that with this book, the reader will have a complete guide of prevention, diagnosis and treatment of the most serious and common complications after STF injections.

For practical purposes, flow charts are provided according to the principal clinical finding and the product injected (HA, CaHA, PLLA or non-resorbable fillers). Therapeutic approaches are outlined in the step-wise treatment algorithms that are based on published articles, as well clinical experience of the authors. These guidelines are not intended to be complete but should be regarded as a basis for treatment and discussion by aesthetic clinicians.

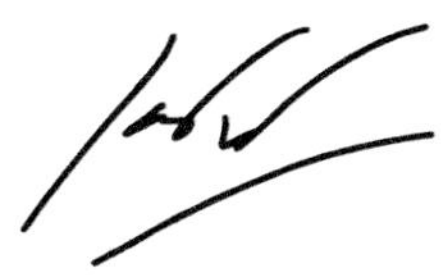

Jani van Loghem, MD PhD
Founder UMA Institute
academy@uma-institute.com

01

avoiding and minimizing complications

Jani van Loghem, MD PhD
Ruscha Wijdeveld

introduction

In this chapter we discuss different variables that influence the risk of complications after soft tissue filler (SFT) injections: the patient, the products and the physician (instruments, techniques, knowledge of anatomy and of complication management).

Patient history

Individual anatomy, asymmetries in anatomy, scars, medication, supplements, allergies and the patient's immune system all influence the a-priori risk of developing STF complications. For many complications, clear recommendations are given to minimize risk for development of these complications.

Product choice

Various product characteristics like color, reversibility, rheological properties, cross linking techniques and immune stimulation are discussed. Choosing the most appropriate product for specific indications will reduce risks of developing complications.

Anatomy

Knowledge of the arterial anatomy is of the utmost importance in order to reduce risk of vascular complications. In-depth medical training is necessary as well as continuing medical education to brush up the anatomical knowledge of the injector in order to avoid delicate structures.

Techniques

Choosing the safest techniques is dependent on the anatomy; the location of important structures as well as the direction of arteries. Aspiration as a safety test has high specificity, but low sensitivity, making this safety test of low value with negative test results (no blood in the needle hub). Cannulas seem safer than needles, as they are less likely to enter into a blood vessel. They are also more precise when predicting the anatomical layer in which the filler is injected.

The 10 safety suggestions are given to avoid vascular adverse events.

prevention

Generally, three main factors influence the occurrence of complications: patient, product, and practitioner. The patient's influential characteristics include their medical history, such as genetics, underlying diseases, coagulation status, previous surgery and scars, allergies and use of medication. Product-related complications have to do with product characteristics like color, immune stimulatory properties, hygroscopic properties and rheologic properties. Practitioner, or injection technique-related, complications have to do with knowledge of anatomy, (wrongful) product choice, the instruments (needle vs cannula, injection device), the technical approach (e.g., injection depth, injection speed and injection volume), and lastly the experience of the physician, including the knowledge of managing complications should they arise.

Unfortunately, complications cannot be avoided 100%. Even if the injector has the best products and safest techniques, the risk of complications is never zero. To minimize risks and severity of complications however, specific variables should be considered: knowledge of anatomy (medical training), patient characteristics, injection techniques, instruments and materials, the chosen product and needle or cannula. Lastly, the injector should know how to react if a complication arises. Knowledge of the algorithms in this book is a valuable tool to prevent serious AEs.

1.1 Patient history

Of the triad of factors determining the a-priori risk of soft tissue filler (STF) complications, the injector has the least influence on the patient. The injector must always remember that individual anatomy varies, also between left and right sides, and that the patient's specific anatomy is more likely to be different than the same as in the anatomy books. Taking a good patient history is important in determining risk factors. Especially rhinoplasty and other surgical procedures can change anatomy and induce scar formation and fibrotic tissue. Even when using non-traumatic cannulas, a post-surgical area can be very difficult to get through, forcing the injector to use force, thus increasing the risk to penetrate an arterial wall with the cannula.

Ask the patient about ease of bruising and if with previous treatments there was significant bruising. If so, a slower approach during the treatment could be considered. Ask about edema, after previous treatments and normally occurring edema in the morning. This could affect product choice (e.g., less hygroscopic products). Ask about previous post inflammatory hyperpigmentation, for example after a small wound like a pimple; this could affect the choice of needle vs cannula as well as the post treatment advice. Ask about medication, especially inform about immunosuppressives (risk of infection and biofilm) and anticoagulants (like aspirine, warfarine, dipyridamol, clopidogrel, NSAIDs, fish oil, vitamin E, ginko biloba, ginseng, etc.).

The patient's immune system is important in the formation of late inflammatory reactions. The type of Human Leucocyte Antigen (HLA) complex is thought to play a role in the likelihood of late inflammatory complications such as granuloma formation. Therefore, it's important to inquire about allergies, to get a general idea of how reactive the patient is to various allergens. Furthermore, there are some patients allergic to lidocaine and because lidocaine is integrated in most filler products, care should be taken not to inject those into patients with a known allergy to lidocaine. An overview of preventive measure is depicted in Table 1 for when a-priori risks are increased in patients.

> Prevention is about the 3 Ps: Patient, Product and Provider. We have to study all the variables that influence complication risks prior to treatment.

Table 1
Complications and adverse events and their preventative measures

Complications and adverse events	Prevention
Pain on injection	Local anesthesia, starting on the left side
Ecchymosis and hematomas	Cold packs, adrenalized lidocaine, use of blunt cannulas. Beware of patients on anticoagulants, and perform immediate compression when visible bleeding is seen
Neovascularization	Place fillers only subcutaneously (not in the skin), beware of patients with rosacea
Hyperpigmentation	Beware of patients with Fitzpatrick skin types V / VI, and of sun exposure after bruising/hematoma
Tyndall effect	Select the correct filler, avoid superficial filler placement
Postinterventional edema	Split treatment over multiple visits, beware of patients with rosacea who have increased risk of erythema and edema after treatment.
Malar edema	No superficial injections in the area of the malar septum, beware of personal or family history of malar edema
Allergic reaction	Beware of patients with history of allergic reactions, consider performing a skin test
Non-inflammatory nodules	Proper injection technique, product choice and selection of target area, avoid overcorrection
Inflammatory nodules	Provide an aseptic working environment, avoid products with higher risk of granuloma formation
Infection	Provide an aseptic working environment, use only high quality products (prophylactic antibiotics/antivirals)
Vascular compromise (necrosis, blindness)	Use blunt cannulas (25G or thicker) and small boluses in high-risk areas, slow injection, long aspiration (needle), manual compression of arteries. Beware of post-surgical patients (scars).
Migration of filler	Proper product selection

product choice

1.2 Product choice

Product-related complications can be visible product, palpable product (nodule), reaction to the product ((allergy, discoloration, late inflammatory reaction) and edema. Specific product characteristics will determine the choice of the injector, being rheological properties, hygoscopic properties, monophasic or biphasic product, color and reversibility.

Visible or palpable product after injection can be prevented by not injecting too superficial or injecting a product that is designed for superficial injections, like a low viscosity, low elasticity, highly cohesive product. Choosing a transparent product like an hyaluronic acid (HA) will reduce risk of visible depositions compared to colored products (like calcium hydroxylapatite (CaHA) which is colored white) on superficial injections. Other discolorations like the Tyndall effect can be avoided by injecting a non-transparent product, as such a product will not result in an optic chamber with its absorption of red light and reflection of blue light. Some products with high elasticity and cohesivity have more tendency to accumulate in mobile areas with significant muscular activity, like around the modiolus or in the lips. These products may have an increased risk of nodule formation.

To avoid edema and puffiness, a product that does not attract a lot of water should be chosen. When a patient requires a sharp definition (compared to a rounder result) like in male aesthetics or when reshaping the jawline in women, a product with low hygoscopic properties like CaHA should be chosen. For areas like the infraorbital area, with high a-priori risk of edema, a low HA concentration should be chosen.

To reduce risk of late inflammatory reactions, a product that is most similar to the human form should be chosen. In the world of HA, that means a monophasic non (or low) cross-linked product. When HA molecules are crosslinked, what essentially happens is that the three-dimensional shape of the HA is changed. This results in a longer half-time as the patient's hyaluronidase cannot reach the target sites as easily, but it also results in a conformational change that could activate an immune response. Particle-based biphasic gels could contain particles with a spikey surface, resulting in higher risk of late reactions. Smooth surfaces are known to have much reduced risk of late immune reactions. CaHA seems to have the lowest risk of late inflammatory reactions among all soft tissue filler products on the market.[2]

1.3 Anatomy

Lastly, there are the practitioner-related complications. A thorough understanding of the facial anatomy is critical before you start treating patients. Especially for the avoidance of vascular complications, anatomical knowledge of the arterial system is of the utmost importance. In-depth medical training is therefore necessary as well as continuing medical education to brush up the knowledge of the injector. If an STF is injected into an artery, both peripheral and retinal ischemia could result from this embolization, possibly resulting in tissue necrosis and/or blindness. Blindness is considered to be the most severe complication after STF injection. And even though there are anecdotal reports of patients regaining vision, treatment options in the acute phase are limited and avoidance is most important. When injecting in a specific facial area, the injector should know at least the two following variables:

01 Risk level of blindness of the area

02 Depth and direction of the relevant arteries

Based on these two factors, the injector should choose a specific approach, always bearing in mind that there is a great variation in arterial anatomy.

The general direction of the arteries is important to know, because it has implications for the choice of entry point when using non-traumatic cannulas (Figure 1). As we have learnt from our cadaver dissections, entering a cannula into an artery is shockingly easy, especially for the smaller gauge cannulas like the 27G cannulas.[3] But also a 22G cannula can easily be inserted into an artery of a cadaver head. There are just two main conditions: the artery has to be relatively fixed in its surrounding tissue (like in scar tissue, or in the area of neurovascular bundles) and it has to be parallel to the cannula.[3] If these two conditions are met, the cannula can easily be inserted into the artery. Apart from direction, an understanding of arterial depth is important (Table 2).

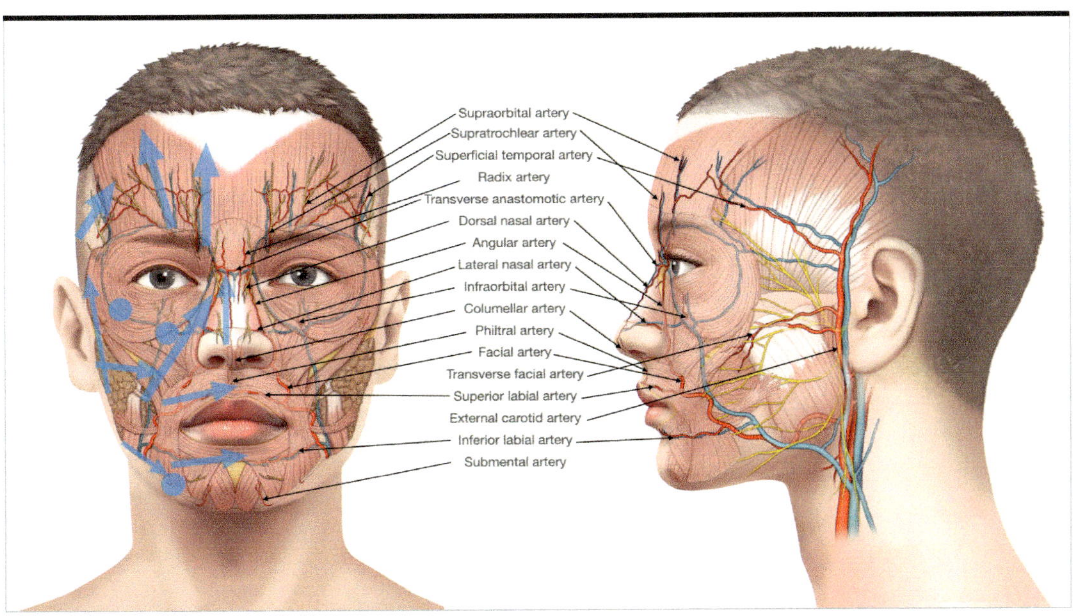

Figure 1
Arterial anatomy: general direction of arteries

Schematic representation of the general direction of the main arteries (blue arrows) and foramina (blue circles).

Choke vessels

In detailed study of flaps in the 1980s performed by G.I. Taylor et al, the researchers observed some fine vessels which they later named 'choke vessels'[189]. Choke vessels are important for the study of vascular occlusion after the injection of soft tissue fillers. Previous research by H. Jajoria et al.[190] showed that choke vessels connect adjacent angiosomes. According to Brodmann (2013)[191], angiosomes are generally understood to be an anatomic tissue unit (consisting of skin, subcutaneous tissue, fascia, muscle, and bone) that is supplied by a source artery and drained by veins.[191]

Choke vessels normally experience minimal blood flow due to opposing pressure from adjacent vascular networks.[189] They may dilate and become active when increased blood flow is required, such as when vascular occlusion occurs in one of the adjacent vascular trees. In the latter case a perforator vessel can successfully perfuse an adjacent vascular territory via dilation of a choke vessel.[192]

Causes for vascular occlusion after filler injections are external vascular compression (which is still under debate), vascular spasm and intravascular embolism.[66] Some dermal fillers may elicit an active intravascular inflammatory response when injected intravascularly, resulting in increased levels of vascular obstruction. Even though hyaluronic acid fillers are well tolerated in connective tissue [193] they are highly inflammatory when injected intra-arterially. Unlike other vessels, choke vessels can respond with spasm, reducing blood flow and diffusion of the filler into bordering vascular angiosomes.[190] The spasm of the vessel prevents the filler from spreading into the adjacent vascular angiosomes and is causing more ischemia that eventually may lead to necrosis.[193]

Other fillers (such as CaHA-based fillers), which elicit less or no inflammatory response when injected intra-arterially, cause less spasm, allowing the filler to spread over a larger vascular network. When low doses of these fillers are injected intra-arterially, they can remain subclinical because they have spread and diluted significantly.

We believe that when filler is injected intravascularly, hyaluronic acid may do more damage in low doses as the intravascular HA may cause vascular spasm, distant to the obstructing embolus and thus widen the area of hypoxemia. However, in certain situations, non-hyaluronic acid fillers may do more damage in higher doses as a larger area spread over multiple angiosomes may become ischemic, as the filler can more freely spread to adjacent angiosomes.

Table 2

The most important arteries in the face with their expected anatomical layer (based on Mendelson's 5-layer classification: 1: skin; 2: subcutaneous; 3: musculo-aponeurotic; 4: retaining ligaments and spaces; 5: periosteum and deep fascias) and their expected general direction. Note: anatomic variation is very common in arterial anatomy. IFS: inferior frontal septum; MFS: middle frontal septum; UFS: upper frontal septum. (Table taken from Van Loghem *et al.*[3].)

Artery	Expected anatomical layer	Expected direction
Supratrochlear a.	Below the IFS: Level 2-5 Between IFS and MFS: Level 2-3 Above UFS: Level 2	Vertical
Supraorbital a.	Below the IFS: Level 2-5 Between IFS and MFS: Level 2-3 Above UFS: Level 2	Vertical with the lateral branch diagonal
Superficial temporal a.	Level 3	Parietal branch: vertical Frontal branch: diagonal
Deep temporal a. (anterior and posterior)	Level 5	Vertical
Dorsal nasal a.	Level 2	Vertical
Lateral nasal a.	Level 2	Around the ala (vertical to horizontal)
Columellar a.	Level 2	Vertical
Angular a.	Level 2	Vertical
Facial a.	Below zygomaticus mm: level 4 Above zygomaticus mm: level 2	Below mandible: horizontal Between mandible and ala: diagonal
External carotid a.	Level 4	Vertical
Transverse facial a.	Level 4 lateral Level 2 medial	Horizontal
Superior labial a.	Level 4	Horizontal
Inferior labial a.	Level 4	Lateral: horizontal; Medial: vertical
Submental artery	Level 4	Below mandible: horizontal At mentum: vertical
Infraorbital a.	Level 4-5	Diagonal, horizontal and vertical branches
Zygomaticofacial a.	Level 4-5	Diagonal, horizontal and vertical branches
Mental a.	Level 4-5	Diagonal, horizontal and vertical branches

1.4 Injection technique

The injection technique used is probably the most important factor that determines the risk of complications. There are several preventative measures that can be taken, summarized in the list below (taken from Van Loghem *et al.*[3,4]).

01 Use blunt cannulas with a gauge of 25G or thicker (if the injector is comfortable with cannulas)

02 Choose the anatomical layer with the lowest risk of arterial presence

03 Choose a cannula direction as perpendicular to the artery as possible

04 To pass a fascia, ligament or other expected resistance, some force is allowed

05 After reaching the desired anatomical layer, no force should be used ('tea-time technique') Where the syringe is lightly held between two or three fingers

06 When the cannula tip reaches a resistance, a gentle, back and forth motion, combined with a rolling technique (the 'pencil-rolling technique') should be used to pass resistances without using force

07 Take extra care near neuromuscular bundles, scars and other areas where arteries are surrounded with dense tissue that may prevent the artery from being pushed aside

08 Around the supratrochlear and dorsal nasal arteries, use the non-dominant thumb and index finger to press on the nasion to temporarily block blood flow (and prevent embolus displacement)". See Figure 2.

09 Inject low volumes (0.025 ml or less per retrograde linear thread) in the high risk periocular area to reduce the chance of reaching the central retinal artery (the JVL Bolus)

10 Inject slowly to reduce chances of retrograde displacement of the embolus against the blood flow of the ophthalmic artery branches in the high risk periocular area

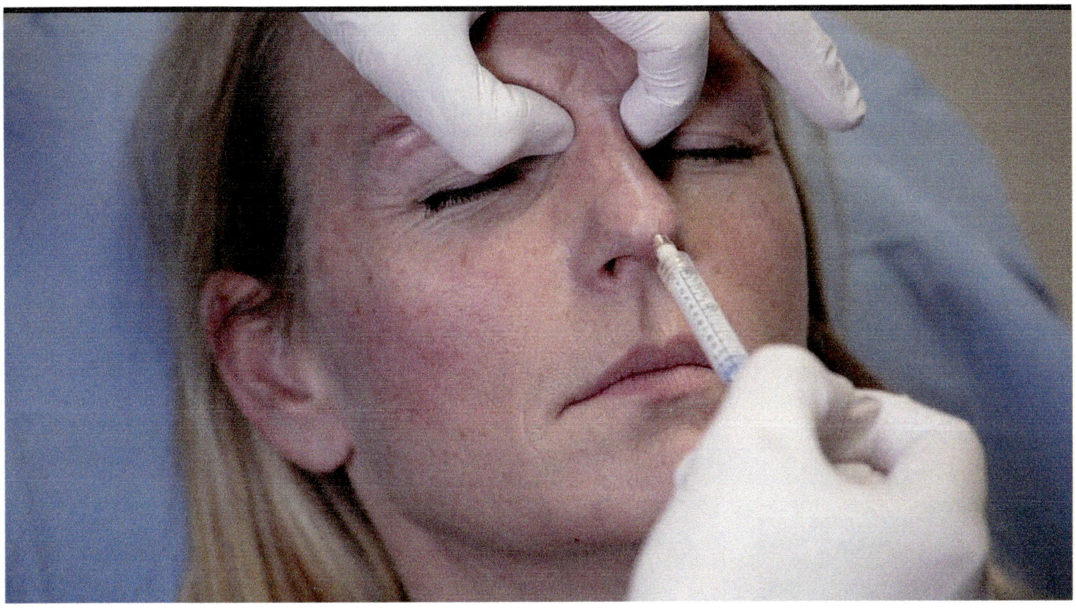

Figure 2

While the injecting hand injects a maximum of 0.025 ml per retrograde linear thread, the fingers of the non-injecting hand press on the nasion, thereby compressing and temporarily stopping blood flow of the supratrochlear artery, the dorsal nasal artery and their connecting arteries in that area. A potential arterial embolus in one of these arteries won't be able to be pushed beyond this point of manual arterial closure.

To avoid serious vascular AEs, the most important recommendation is to inject small amounts of filler per bolus or retrograde. Even though the chance of hitting an artery increases with the number of times the needle is advanced in the tissue, the chances of devastating sequelae is reduced with smaller amounts of fillers injected into an artery. Blindness for example can occur after injecting in the supratrochlear artery. In such case, the filler travels through the vessel towards the ophthalmic artery until it reaches the bifurcation of the central retinal artery branching off the ophthalmic artery where it can embolize the retina and cause blindness. To cover that distance, the volume necessary is somewhere between 0.04 and 0.12 ml.[6] If a maximum injection volume of 0.025 is chosen (the so-called JVL Bolus), the chance of blinding the patient is drastically reduced to next to zero.

The number of dermal punctures is also relevant. The more the amount of needle punctures, the (exponentially) higher the risk of infection and/or biofilm formation.[7] Using non-traumatic cannulas, the number of dermal punctures is lower than when using needles, but a no-touch handling should be done and extra care should be taken when maneuvering the often long cannula close to the patient's hair, the non-sterile swabs or the patient's clothes, as contamination could result in the formation of biofilm as well as infections.

needle vs. cannula

1.5 Needle vs. cannula

Although the opinions differ, most clinicians nowadays agree that cannulas pose a smaller risk of complications. It was shown that higher number of skin penetrations exponentially increased the chance of biofilm formation.[7]
As abovementioned, fewer entry points (when using blunt cannulas) reduce the risk of infection and biofilm. Besides, in an observational cadaver study, it was shown that because of back-flow through the tunnel that was made with a needle, product was not only injected on the periosteum, which was the target depth, but also travelled retrogradely along the needle and ended up in various anatomical levels. This was a consistent finding in five facial areas and a careful conclusion can therefore be made that this is a general observation describing what happens using a needle for STF injection. When the injector uses a needle, generally, the needle is advanced (almost) perpendicularly to the skin and advanced to the periosteum. Then, when the needle is in contact with the periosteum, the injector starts injecting. The product then starts flowing out of the needle into the deep tissue and will logically start following the path of least resistance. Part of the product will flow back along the needle trajectory, as the needle has just created a pathway by being advanced. In some areas that could be exactly what the injector wants: creating pillars of filler, like in the chin or cheeks. In other areas, like the forehead, the injector wants to be certain that the filler remains in a specific anatomical level because of the depth localization of important arteries.

If an injector is more comfortable with a needle, than that is probably the safest instrument to choose. If the injector is comfortable with both, the cannula probably has lower risk of vascular events, irregularities and bruising.

1.6. Aspiration

Aspiration is often listed as a prevention measure, but there are many variables that contribute to the sensitivity of aspiration.[8] Apart from needle diameter and length, extrusion and aspiration of STFs are dependent on differences in physiochemical structure and rheological properties. The elastic quantitative measurement (elasticity) of a STF's stiffness and its ability to resist deformation under applied pressure are known as G prime (G').[9] The higher the G' of a STF, the less it will deform under pressure and the more stored energy it retains. Thickness, or viscosity of a STF in its fluid form (η^*), refers to the measure of its resistance to gradual reformation by shear stress and how it flows from the needle while being injected. Therefore, elasticity and viscosity will also determine how a STF product behaves in the lumen of the needle when aspiration is applied. The higher the G' and η^*, the more force is needed to obtain a positive aspiration result by emptying a needle filled with STF material. Most commercial STF products have a viscosity between 7.307 centipoises (cP) (Juvederm Ultra, Allergan Inc., Irvine, CA, USA) and 349 830 cP (Radiesse, Merz Pharmaceuticals GmbH, Frankfurt, Germany).[10] When comparing these values to water (0.890 cP at 25°C) and blood (between 3.000 and 4.000 cP at 37°C), it becomes clear that the results of an aspiration test may not always be reliable as the high viscosity of STFs would mean that a very high suction pressure must be applied in order to obtain a positive aspiration test result.[11] An overview of the aspiration results are shown in Table 3.[8]

aspiration

Table 3
Aspiration test result
Courtesy of Van Loghem *et al.*[8]

● Positive (within 1 second)
○ Positive (between 1 and 10 seconds)
◍ False-negative (when still negative after 10 seconds)
RL: Ringer's Lactate; EDTA: Ethylenediaminetetraacetic acid

Digits in circles indicate seconds

Product	**Agent**	**Needle**										
		Gauge (G)	**23**	**25**		**27**			**28**	**29**	**30**	**33**
		Length (mm)	**19**	**13**	**25**	**12**	**13**	**20**	**19**		**12**	**13**	**13**
Control (Saline)	RL + ink		●	●			●		●			●	●
	Blood + EDTA		●	●			●		●			●	●
Belotero Hydro	RL + ink		●	●			●		●			●	⑥
	Blood + EDTA		●	●			●		●			●	⑨
Belotero Soft	RL + ink		●	●			●		●			●	⑤
	Blood + EDTA		●	●			●		●			●	④
Belotero Balance	RL + ink		●	③			●		◍			●	◍
	Blood + EDTA		●	③			⑤		◍			⑦	◍
Belotero Intense	RL + ink		⑧	⑧			③		◍			◍	◍
	Blood + EDTA		⑨	⑥			⑤		◍			◍	◍
Belotero Volume	RL + ink		●	●			②		◍			◍	◍
	Blood + EDTA		●	⑤			⑧		◍			◍	◍
Radiesse 0.8 (undiluted)	RL + ink		◍	◍			◍		◍			◍	◍
	Blood + EDTA		◍	◍			◍		◍			◍	◍
Radiesse 0.8 (diluted)	RL + ink		●	●			●		◍			③	◍
	Blood + EDTA		●	●			●		◍			◍	◍
Radiesse 1.5 (undiluted)	RL + ink		④	⑥			⑧		◍			◍	◍
	Blood + EDTA		◍	◍			◍		◍			◍	◍
Radiesse 1.5 (diluted)	RL + ink		●	●			●		◍			⑤	◍
	Blood + EDTA		⑦	③			③		◍			◍	◍
Radiesse Plus 1.5	RL + ink		④	③			④	⊖	◍			◍	◍
	Blood + EDTA		⑥	③			⑥	⊖	◍			◍	◍
Etermis 2	RL + ink		●	●			●	●	●		●	●	⑤
	Blood + EDTA		●	●			●	●	●		●	●	⑧
Etermis 3	RL + ink		●	●		●	●		◍			③	◍
	Blood + EDTA		●	●		●	●		◍			③	◍

Continued on next page

aspiration

Product	Agent	Needle										
		Gauge (G)	**23**	**25**		**27**			**28**	**29**	**30**	**33**
		Length (mm)	**19**	**13**	**25**	**12**	**13**	**20**	**19**		**12**	**13**	**13**
Etermis 4	RL + ink		●	●	●	●	●		○			③	○
	Blood + EDTA		●	●	③	●	●		○			④	○
Juvéderm Volbella	RL + ink		●	●			●		●			●	④
	Blood + EDTA		●	●			●		●			●	⑥
Juvéderm Volift	RL + ink		●	●			●		●			●	④
	Blood + EDTA		●	●			●		●			●	⑤
Juvéderm Voluma	RL + ink		●	●			●		○			○	○
	Blood + EDTA		●	●			●		○			○	○
Juvéderm Ultra 2	RL + ink		⑤	⑤			③		○			○	○
	Blood + EDTA		⑨	⑧			④		○			○	○
Juvéderm Ultra 3	RL + ink		④	③			②		○			○	○
	Blood + EDTA		④	④			③		○			○	○
Juvéderm Ultra 4	RL + ink		○	⑦			⑥		○			○	○
	Blood + EDTA		○	⑩			⑩		○			○	○
Juvéderm Ultra Smile	RL + ink		④	②			②		○			⑦	○
	Blood + EDTA		⑩	③			③		○			○	○
Restylane Kysse	RL + ink		⑥	●			②		○			○	○
	Blood + EDTA		○	③			③		○			○	○
Restylane Defyne	RL + ink		⑨	⑩			⑦		○			②	⑧
	Blood + EDTA		○	○			○		○			○	○
Restylane Refyne	RL + ink		⑥	④			④		○			③	⑨
	Blood + EDTA		○	⑤			⑧		○			○	○
Restylane Lyft	RL + ink		●	②			②		⑧	④		○	○
	Blood + EDTA		●	○			○		○	④		○	○
Restylane Lidocaine	RL + ink		●	●			●		●	●		②	⑧
	Blood + EDTA		●	●			●		●	●		○	○
Restylane Vylume	RL + ink		⑦	⑥			⑦		○			⑦	○
	Blood + EDTA		⑨	⑦			⑦		○			○	○
Restylane Fynesse	RL + ink		●	●			●		⑧			③	⑥
	Blood + EDTA		●	●			●		○			④	⑧

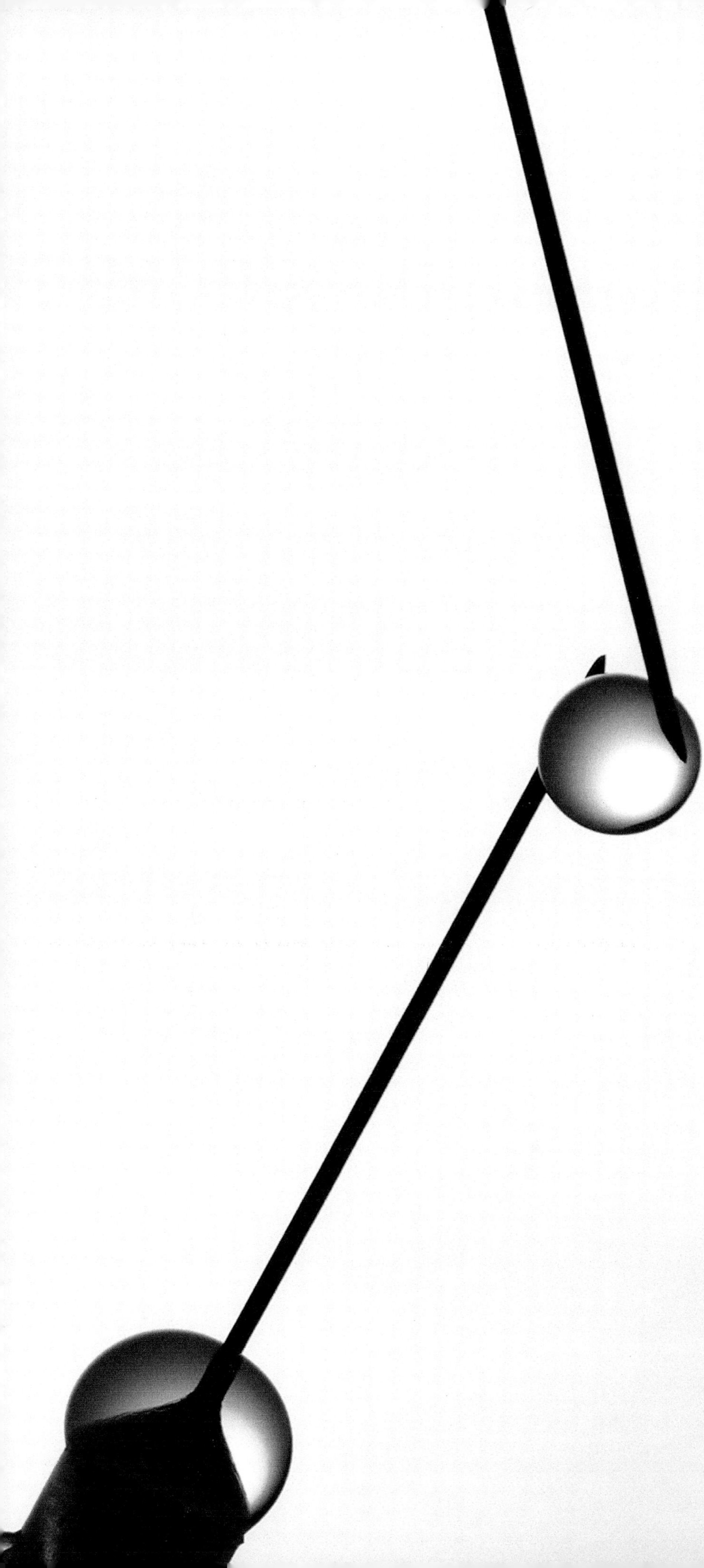

02
HA, CaHA and PLLA complication management

Philippe Snozzi, MD
Jani van Loghem, MD PhD
Pieter Siebenga, MD PhD
Job Thuis, MD
Fred Tjan, MD
Rebecca Fitzgerald, MD
Ruscha Wijdeveld

introduction

In this chapter we will cover clinical presentations of soft tissue filler induced complications. We will be sharing comprehensive algorithms as a guide to approach the most common soft tissue filler complications:

- skin discoloration
- edema
- infection
- nodules
- vascular compromise (peripheral and central)

We have included both hyaluronic acid (HA) as well as calcium hydroxylapatite (CaHA, Radiesse) in these algorithms and have chosen to base the management strategy on clinical presentation rather than final diagnosis of the complication in order to make the algorithms practical. Management of poly-L-lactic acid (PLLA, Sculptra) is discussed separately in this chapter and management of non-resorbable filler complications will be discussed in the next chapter.

skin discoloration

2.1 Skin discoloration (ecchymosis, hematoma, Tyndall effect)

Skin discoloration is a natural phenomenon directly after injection, where there will be some redness. Other significant skin discolorations may also occur at the site of treatment, which, depending on the type of discoloration, is usually mild in intensity, self-limiting and usually resolves within a few days to weeks. The main categories of skin discoloration complications include hematoma/ecchymosis (bruising), neovascularization, hyperpigmentation, and the Tyndall effect/brightening. Ischemia will be discussed later (see chapter Vascular Compromise). Each of these complications has differing times to onset, clinical presentation, and differential diagnoses (Figure 3).

Figure 3

Skin Discoloration (Differential Diagnosis)

Skin Discoloration (Differential Diagnosis)

Diagnosis	Hematoma	Neovascularisation	Hyperpigmentation	Tyndall effect/Skin brightening/visible product	Ischemia
Time of occurrence	• Within minutes to hours	• Within days to weeks	• Within days to weeks	• Within days	See Vascular Compromise Section
Clinical presentation	• Deep hematoma may appear as a subacute swelling, with no visible bruises • Temporary or permanent hemosiderin deposits are possible	• Telangiectasia days to weeks after intradermal filler treatment • Often in the upper nasolabial fold region	• Post-inflammatory hyperpigmentation • Especially with Fitzpatrick skin types IV-VI	• HA: blue coloration / lighter skin • CaHA: yellow discoloration	
Differential diagnosis	• Erythema (several possibilities) • Ischemia (blue-gray phase) • Post-inflammatory hyperpigmentation	• Rosacea	• Hemosiderin deposits	• (Malar) edema	
Therapy	• Heparin- or Vit. K - containing ointment • IPL • Hemosiderin deposits: alpha hydroxy acid, or laser	• Mostly self limiting in 3 - 12 months without therapy • Laser • IPL	• Sun protection SP50 • Bleaching agent • Chemical peels • IPL (skin type I-IV) • Nd:YAG laser (Skin type V-VI)	• HA: inject Hyaluronidase • CaHA: expression	
Prophylaxis	• Apply immediate compression when visible bleeding is seen • Use blunt cannulas • Beware of patients using oral anticoagulants	• By placing fillers only subcutaneous (cannula) • Increased risk in rosacea patients possible	• By placing fillers only subcutaneous (cannula) • Beware skin type Fitzpatrick V / VI	• Selecting the right filler • Avoid too superficial placement of filler	

Based on clinical presentation, these algorithms will aid you in making a clinical diagnosis and in managing the complication.

2.1.1 Bruising

Ecchymosis (bruising) is the most common localized event and can occur in up to 68% of patients.[12] It can occur after injection with all STFs. The dermal and subdermal anatomical planes are more prone to bruising than the deep planes (e.g., supraperiosteal).[13] Formation of larger hematomas are less common and usually occur within minutes or hours due to inadvertent laceration of facial arterial vessels. Rather than forming a bruise, if blood beneath the superficial fascia becomes trapped, a firm mass can appear.

To minimize the risk of hematoma formation, all anticoagulant and antiplatelet medication (e.g., aspirin, warfarin, dabigatran, etc.) or potentially blood thinning supplements (e.g., fish oil, vitamin E, St. John's Wort, ginseng, etc.) should be temporarily discontinued.[14] However, anticoagulation or antiplatelet therapy should never be discontinued without the consultation with the treating physician, especially in patients with a high cardiovascular risk profile. Epinephrine inhibits the activation of eosinophils that play a role in bruising and causes vasoconstriction. When adrenalized lidocaine is mixed with fillers it may reduce the risk of bruising. Also, blunt cannulas are less likely to result in bruising compared to sharp needles.[3,15,16] When sharp needles are used, use small gauge needles, slow injection of small aliquots, and limit the number of transcutaneous puncture sites.[7,17]

In case of bruising, compression should be applied immediately when bleeding is suspected. When there is evidence of a hematoma, compression for a few minutes is advised. Cold compresses may be used to reduce edema and promote vasoconstriction. However, as coagulant proteins have their optimum function at normal body temperature, lowering the temperature may also increase coagulation time. Bruises and hematomas usually resolve spontaneously over several weeks. Patients should be advised to stay out of the sun for the duration of the bruising to minimize the risk of hyperpigmentation formation. Additional treatment may include vitamin K cream BID for 7 days, or intense pulsed light therapy.[18-20] If there is persistent hemosiderin staining, pulsed-dye or potassium titanyl phosphate (KTP) laser treatment is recommended. These lasers emit their light in a spectrum which is more precisely absorbed by hemoglobin than other colors.[21]

Rarely, a palpable nodule due to fibrosis of the hematoma may persist. Also, hyperpigmentation can occur after bruising, especially when inadequate sun protection screen is applied on sunny days.

skin discoloration

2.1.2 Neovascularization

Neovascularization occurs when new capillaries, arterioles, and/or venules are formed at the site of dermal filler injection. Potential pathophysiological mechanisms are tissue trauma, direct stimulation of angiogenesis through HA breakdown products, or, in the case of telangiectasia, dilatation of tiny dermal veins due to increased tissue pressure after intra-dermal filler injection.[22] Neovascularization can occur days to weeks after the procedure but should fade within 3–12 months without treatment. Calcium hydroxylapatite (CaHA, Radiesse®) has been shown to significantly increase angiogenesis in a histological study.[138] Too superficially placed CaHA may therefor result in visible vascularization that can last beyond weeks to months if not treated. Intense pulsed light and lasers are effective if erythema or telangiectasias do not show spontaneous improvement, with the choice of laser being dependent upon the size of the vessel.[20,21]

2.1.3 Hyperpigmentation

Hyperpigmentation results from either melanin overproduction or the irregular dispersion of melanin (i.e., pigmentary incontinence) following cutaneous inflammation, or residual hemosiderin deposits after bleeding.[23,24] Pigmentary incontinence results from the destruction of the basal cell layer[25], which allows macrophages to accumulate in the upper dermis, where they phagocytose degenerating basal keratinocytes and melanocytes. The release of melanin from these melanocytes is believed to result in hyperpigmentation.[26] Postinflammatory hyperpigmentation (PIH) is a complex process involving both molecular and cellular changes that lead to the overproduction of melanin and/or the irregular dispersion of pigment following inflammation. Mechanistically, the release of prostanoids, cytokines, chemokines and other inflammatory factors is stimulated in PIH.[24] Although PIH can occur in all skin types, it is generally more common among individuals with skin of color, including African Americans, Hispanics/ Latinos, Asians, Native Americans, Pacific Islanders and persons of Middle Eastern descent.[24] A wide range of etiologies has been described, including skin diseases (e.g., acne vulgaris, atopic dermatitis, impetigo, plaque psoriasis and lichen planus); bacterial, fungal and viral infections; allergic reactions; medication-induced PIH; and cutaneous injuries as a result of topical irritants, sunburns and other types of burns, ultraviolet B-induced, and cosmetic procedures.[23,26]

PIH has been reported following HA treatment, with Fitzpatrick skin types IV-VI being more prone to such events.[27,28] However, it is important to distinguish PIH from hemosiderin staining following ecchymosis. First-line treatment of persistent PIH consist of topical cream with hydroquinone (2%-8%), tretinoin and adequate sunscreen. As an alternative one may choose retinol cream. Additional treatment may include chemical peels where a trichloroacetic acid (TCA) 8% to 20% solution have the most optimal results on pigmentations. IPL, a pulsed dye laser or fractional laser also show successful reduction of the hyperpigmentation.

2.1.4 Tyndall effect

Bluish coloration or brightening effects of the skin can occur if HA is injected too superficially or in areas where the overlying skin is thin, such as the tear trough area. This phenomenon, known as the Tyndall effect, is due to partial absorption of red light and reflection of shorter wavelength light (e.g., blue) due to the optic chamber that is formed by a deposition of HA. More superficially placed HA will result in a more severe and longer duration of the Tyndall effect. The Tyndall effect can occur with all HA fillers, but is less likely with certain crosslinking technologies, such as cohesive polydensified matrix (CPM [Belotero Balance]), Vycross (Juvéderm Volbella), and resilient HA (RHA [Teosyal Global Action]), due to the homogeneous tissue integration.[29] Hyaluronidase is the recommended treatment (Figure 4).[20,21,30]

Figure 4

Skin Discoloration (Algorithm)

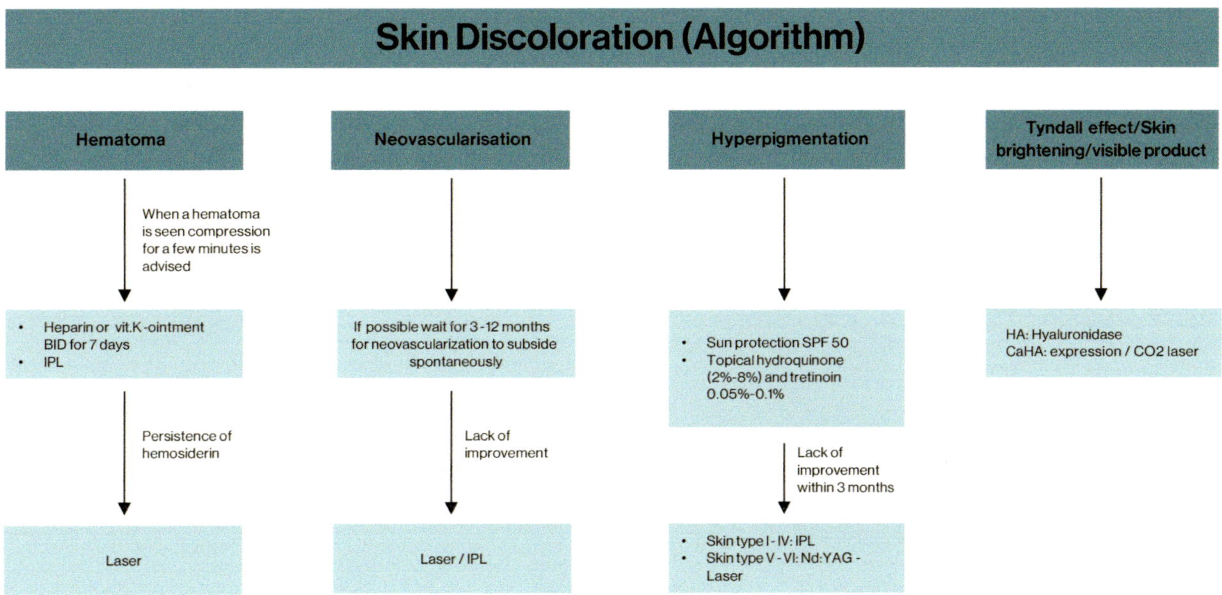

2.1.5 CaHA induced yellowish skin discoloration

Superficial injection of CaHA may result in visible depositions of the product, especially in areas with very thin skin, like the lower eyelids, often combined with erythema. Previously reported therapeutic options are limited and include intralesional triamcinolone, massage, needling, and excision, each with inconsistent results or potential for scarring. Please see the section on treatment of early onset non-inflammatory nodules for treatment or CaHA nodules (chapter 2.4.1). A single session of fractional carbon dioxide (CO_2) laser treatment or 5 sessions of Erbium Yag (1540nm) laser (15 millisecond pulse duration, 8 millijoules, spot size 15 mm, five pulses per treatment over the affected area) may resolve selected cases of superficial CaHA depositions. It was hypothesized that carbon dioxide laser treatment results in high-temperature vaporization of CaHA, with localized melting and rehardening into an alpha-calcium orthophosphate structure that displays increased brittleness with easy cracking and fissuring into multiple pieces.[140] This therapeutic technique may enhance treatment options for superficially placed visible CaHA depositions.

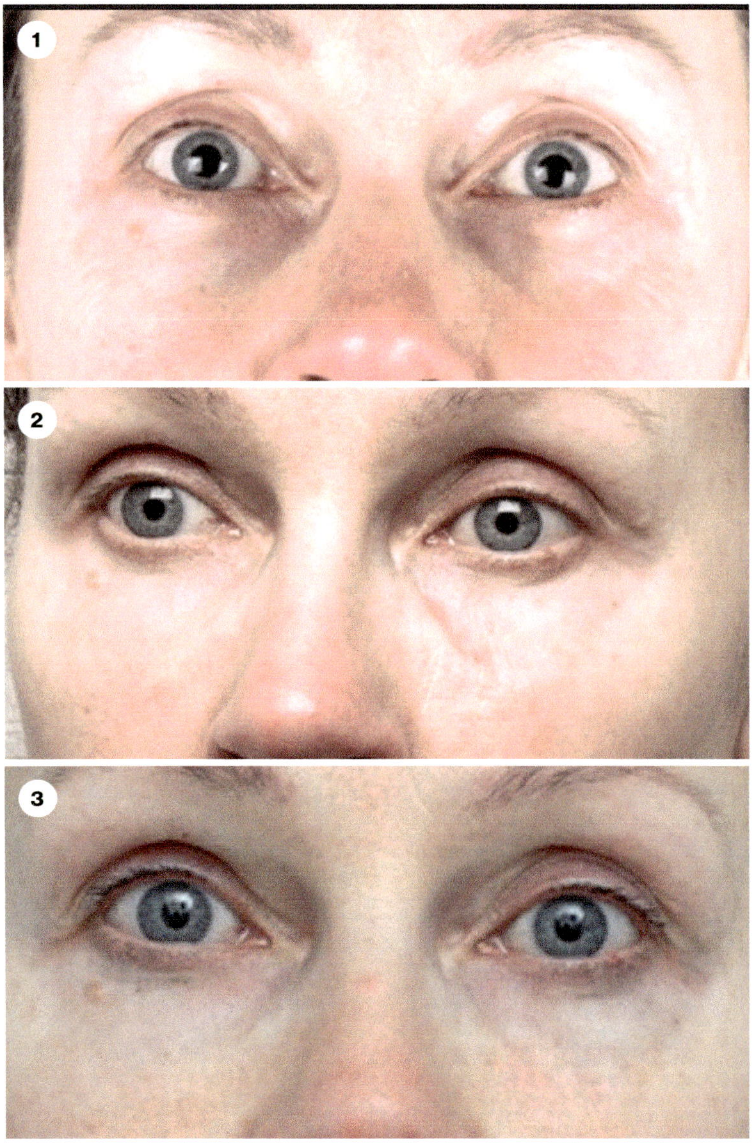

Figure 5
Superficially placed CaHA after scar subcision in a patient with a surgical scar in the left tear trough.

1 Before scar subcision and before hyper diluted CaHA 1:10.
2 Visible CaHA depositions in tear trough 2 months post Tx.
3 Resolution 3 months after after a single session of fractional CO2 laser of the affected area (1 pass of 20%, 4 ms, 10J).

Note skin quality improvement of the lower lid.

2.2 Edema

2.2.1 Edema

A variety of edema types can occur following facial filler treatments: immediate postinterventional edema, histamine-mediated edema, e.g., physical urticaria and immediate type allergy (type I, IgE-mediated), or delayed type allergy (type IV, cell-mediated), and malar edema (Figure 6). These vary in time to occurrence and clinical presentation, and treatment options vary depending upon category (Figure 7).

Figure 6

Anaphylactic Reaction Flow Chart.

Note: print this page to include it in your UMA filler first aid kit

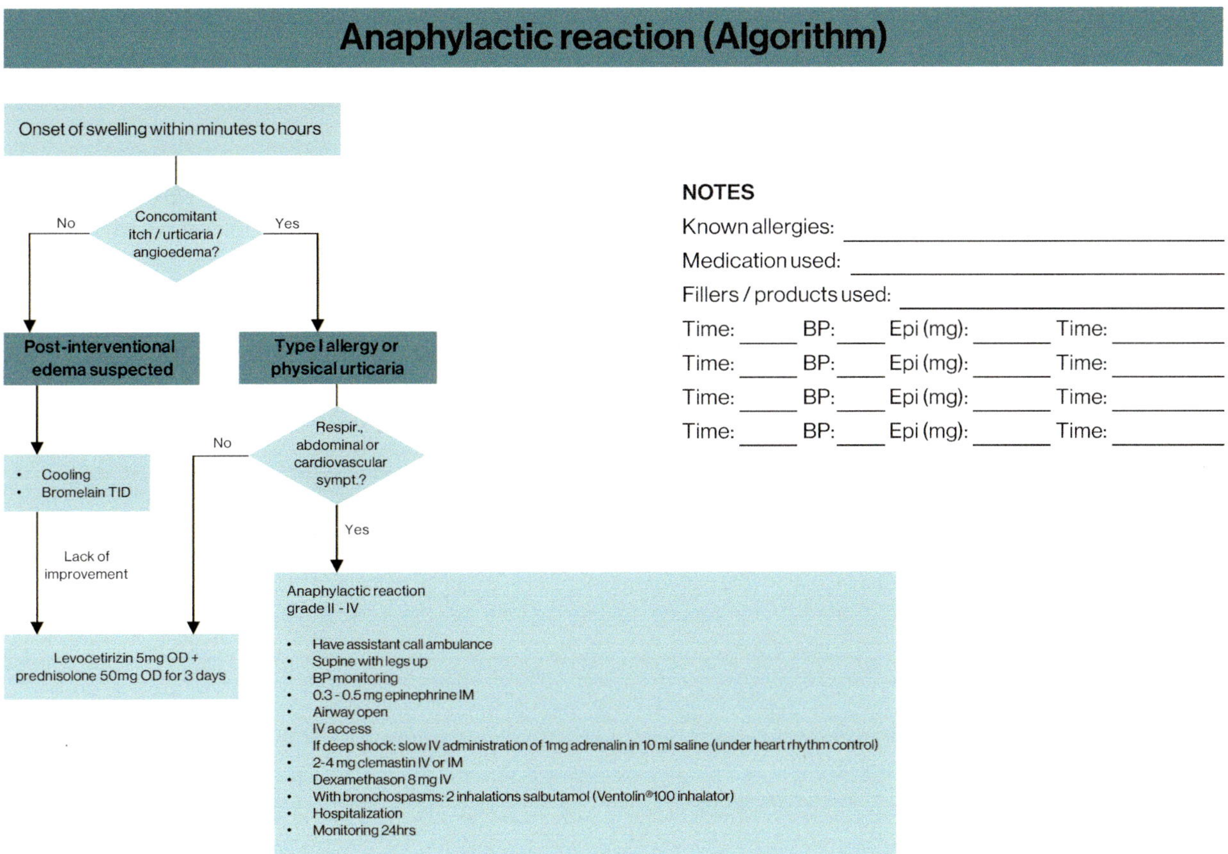

edema

Figure 7
Edema (Algorithm)

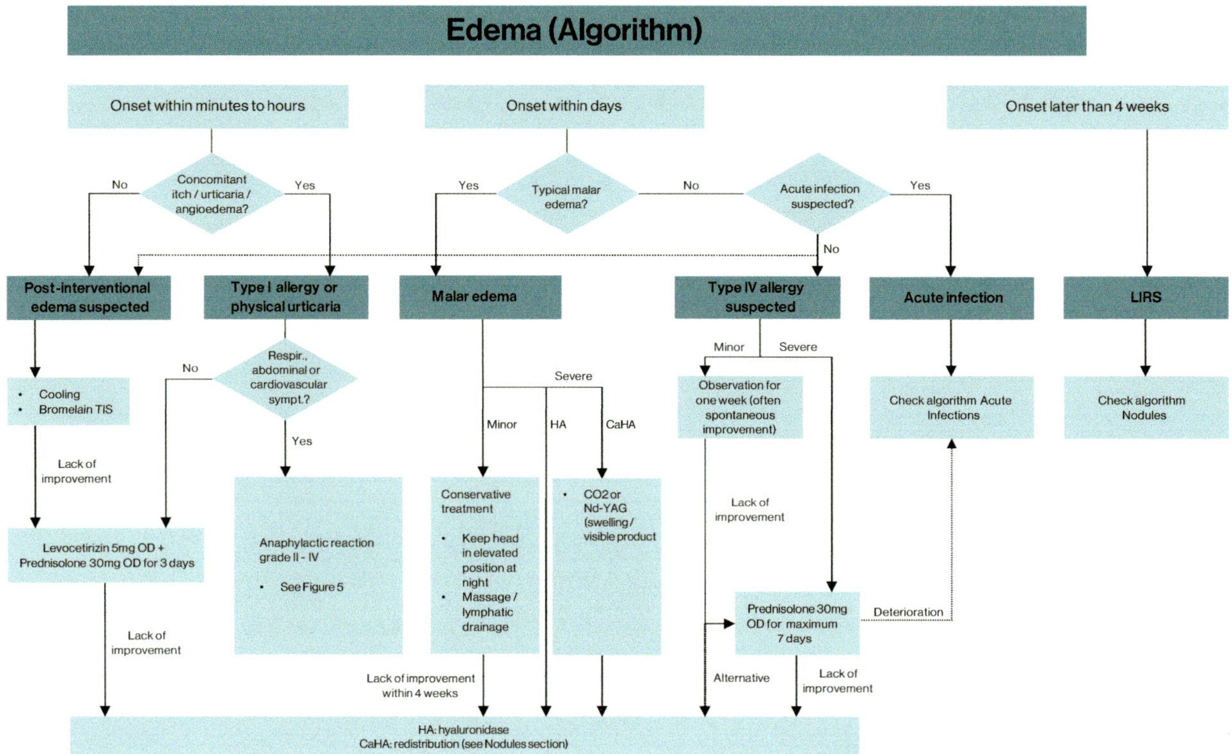

Short-term immediate postintervention edema comprising transient swelling is normal and common to all dermal fillers. It is related to injection volume and technique and usually resolves without medical intervention within 1 week.[20] In severe or persistent cases, bromelain can be prescribed.[20,31]

Some patients may develop histamine-mediated edema, either through direct release of histamine in physical urticaria or through IgE-mediated antibody response from hypersensitivity to components of the filler (type I hypersensitivity reaction).

IgE plays a central role in the pathophysiology of acute allergic reactions and chronic inflammatory allergic diseases. Free IgE in plasma is short-lived and resides for about 1 day, but receptor-bound IgE can remain fixed to cells in tissues for weeks or months. When the antigen is presented (the allergen), IgE stimulate mast cells to degenerate resulting in the release of (among others) pro-inflammatory cytokines, histamine, prostaglandins and proteases. Angioedema occurs within hours after the allergen has been presented to the body. The reaction may be localized, but can also be generalized. Even though type I hypersensitivity reactions are commonly mentioned in literature,[20,21,32] the authors believe that most angioedema cases seen soon after HA injections are due to physical urticaria triggered by mild trauma, rather than IgE-mediated histamine release.[20] Nonetheless, in rare cases, IgE-mediated antibody response to either the disinfection agent (e.g., chlorhexidine) or HA fragments or other filler components (e.g., lidocaine) is possible. Reactions can be severe and long-lasting with either localized or generalized edema. Treatment depends on the severity, but if there is no spontaneous resolution, antihistamines and oral corticosteroids are recommended. Close monitoring is recommended. Firstly, to exclude rapid progression of the angioedema, since this is a medical emergency with a chance of airway obstruction. Secondly, to exclude an infectious etiology that could be causing the edema which would be progressing more slowly. If angioedema occurs after a substantial period of time from the treatment (e.g., months after lip augmentation), it may be due to an acquired angioedema such as drug induced or peri-infectious angioedema , both unrelated to the filler treatment, or LIRS (see chapter 2.4.4).

Delayed hypersensitivity reactions (non-antibody-mediated, type IV) may also occur after dermal filler injection. Typically, the onset will be 1 day (when pre sensitized) to several days after injection, but can be seen as late as several weeks after injection and may persist for many months. Potential triggers are the injection needle in cases of nickel allergy,[33] or possibly residual BDDE and other filler components. Symptoms may include induration, erythema and edema. It is a T lymphocyte mediated reaction rather than due to antibodies. This type of hypersensitivity will not respond to antihistamines. The first choice of treatment will be the removal of the product, in case of HA with hyaluronidase. Adjuvant treatment will involve a short course of oral corticosteroids, laser and/or extrusion until the filler is resorbed.[21,34-36] If the reaction commences more than 3 weeks after injection, late inflammatory response syndrome (LIRS) should be considered (Figure 8).[20]

Figure 8
Malar edema after CaHA injection at 1 week post injection (left and middle) and 2 weeks (right) after injection.

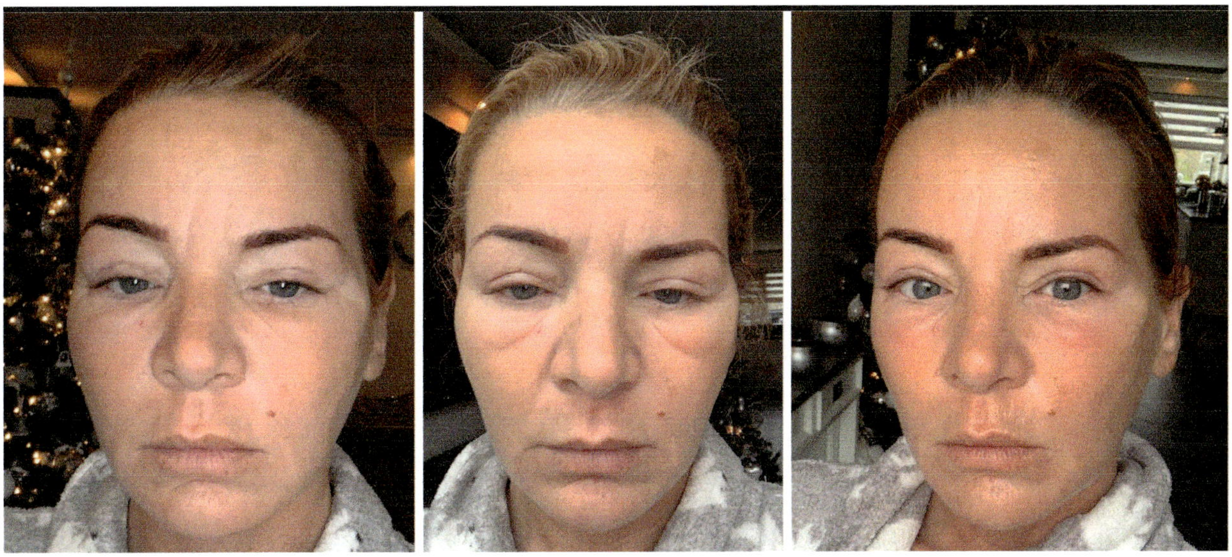

2.2.2 Malar edema

Malar edema is a serious and long-lasting complication that has been reported with all fillers when injected into the infraorbital hollow and tear troughs. Superficial injection of any type of filler is usually the cause of malar edema, but the risk increases with fillers that have a high elasticity and viscosity. This region is particularly susceptible to edema due to an easily compromised lymphatic drainage. Malar edema can occur after compression of the lymphatic vessels trapping lymphatic fluid in between three barriers: the malar septum, the orbicularis retaining ligament (ORL) and the zygomatico-cutaneous ligament (ZCL).[37] Malar edema is difficult to treat, but initial recommendations include lymphatic drainage and massage, with the head elevated at night.[37] In cases of persistent malar edema due to hyaluronic acid injections, hyaluronidase should be administered.[21,37] In case of CaHA induced malar edema, injection of saline followed by Erbium-Yag laser (5 treatments),[139] as well as CO_2 laser (1 treatment)[140] have shown good resolution.

2.3 Infection

The skin is an ecosystem and colonized by a wide range of microorganisms, predominantly by bacteria, but also viruses, fungi, mycobacteria, and protozoa. Most of the time, these microorganisms peacefully coexist with the host, providing protection against foreign invaders and stimulating immune responses if necessary.[39] The skin serves as a barrier to the diverse environment, and, in addition, protects our body from potential assaults by foreign organisms or toxic substances.[39] Disruption of this delicate balance can lead to skin disorders or infections. Skin or soft tissue infections (SSTI) arises when microbes breach the cutaneous surface, especially in patients with skin disorders or diminished local host defenses from conditions such as older age, obesity or HIV, but can also develop after cutaneous trauma (including STF injections). SSTI is a microbial invasion that usually affects the epidermis, dermis, and subcutaneous fat, but may penetrate deeper to the fascial layers and musculotendinous structures.[40] It induces a host response which is typically characterized by rubor, dolor, calor and tumor. These symptoms can be accompanied by fever, suppuration and malaise. If untreated, they can sometimes lead to disseminated infection via the circulatory and lymphatic systems.[41] The most common microorganisms responsible for SSTI include Staphylococcus aureus and/or Streptococci. For abscesses, S. aureus is considered to be the most common pathogen, while Streptococci are the most common cause of cellulitis and erysipelas. They usually have a defined port d'entrée (e.g., entry point of a needle or cannula).[42,43] Necrotizing fasciitis may be monomicrobial or polymicrobial. It is generally caused by S. pyogenes, Vibrio vulnificus, Aeromonas hydrophila, and more recently, MRSA.[38] In fungemia, cutaneous involvement is most often caused by Candida spp., Cryptococcus neoformans, Blastomyces dermatitidis, and Fusarium spp.[44] Candida, Aspergillus, Mucor, and Fusarium species on the other hand are not very common pathogens (Figure 9).[44]

Figure 9

Infections (Differential diagnosis)

Infections (Differential Diagnosis)

Diagnosis	Erysipelas, cellulitis	Abscess	Herpes lesions	Biofilm
Time of occurrence	Acute (within days)			Subacute (within weeks to months)
Suspected culprit	• S. pyogenes, S. aureus • When developing later than two weeks after the injection atypical bacteria may be involved	• S. aureus • When developing later than two weeks after the injection atypical bacteria may be involved	• Herpes Simplex Type I or II	• Pseudomonas species, S. epidermidis, P. acnes, Acinetobacter, others
Clinical presentation	• Sharp (erysipelas) or non-sharply defined (cellulitis) inflammatory swelling • Sometimes fever or malaise • Sometimes lymphadenopathy	• Like cellulitis, but with a palpable, fluctuating mass	• Herpes typical vesicles • Sometimes Lymphadenopathy	See Nodules Section
Differential Diagnosis	• Type IV immune reaction • Edematous granuloma (early onset unusual)	• Cystic granuloma (early onset unusual)	• Vascular compromise (necrosis)	
Diagnostics / Therapy	• Antibiotics • In severe cases, referral to a hospital	• Incision, drainage and culture • Antibiotics • In severe cases, referral to a hospital	• Anti-viral therapy	
Prophylaxis	• Take care to create an aseptic environment during treatments! • Use only high quality products	• Take care to create an aseptic environment during treatments! • Use only high quality products	• Regular history of herpes: valciclovir 500 mg BID for 3 days as a prophylaxis	

As with any procedure that breaches the skin barrier, it is important to maintain a stringent antiseptic treatment area throughout the entire procedure. The patient's skin should be cleansed, and make-up should be removed. Disinfection of a broader area than the treatment area is imperative as there is always the risk of touching untreated skin with the needle or cannula. Disinfection of the skin should be done with chlorhexidine, alcohol, iodine, chloroxylenol or iodophors. The aesthetic physician should remove all jewelry, wash their hands with an antiseptic cleanser, and use gloves.[45] Further, wearing a surgical face mask during the procedure may be considered. Constant vigilance is important, since the syringes are not packaged sterile except the Radiesse syringe. Not touching, and frequently changing, the needle or cannula further reduces infective complications.[7,45] If these necessary hygiene and infection-prevention precautions are taken, then SSTIs are rare.

2.3.1 Acute bacterial infection

Antibiotic therapy is the first line treatment when an acute infection is suspected. Mild cases can successfully be treated with oral broad-spectrum antibiotics. Amoxicillin/clavulanate 625 mg TID or, in the case of a penicillin allergy, clindamycin 600mg TID for 7–10 days is recommended. Unresolved cases or more severe cases require intravenous antibiotics. If possible, specialist infectious disease advice should be sought, and a culture should be obtained to tailor the antibiotic treatment. Abscess formation can occur any time from days to months following treatment. A single abscess is typically the result of contamination through the skin during treatment. However, multiple abscesses are a sign that the contamination occurred in the syringe prior to injection. Abscesses should be treated with incision and drainage and left open for rinsing the wound in the days following. Adjuvant culture-directed antibiotic treatment can be considered. If the abscess emerges late (weeks to months post-injection) and cultures are negative, the abscess may represent a cystic granuloma and should be treated as a late inflammatory reaction (see chapter 2.4 nodules). Removal of the implant should be considered to avoid recurrence of the infection. Injection of hyaluronidase must be done in combination with antibiotic treatment to prevent further spreading of the infection (Figure 10).

Figure 10
Acute Infection

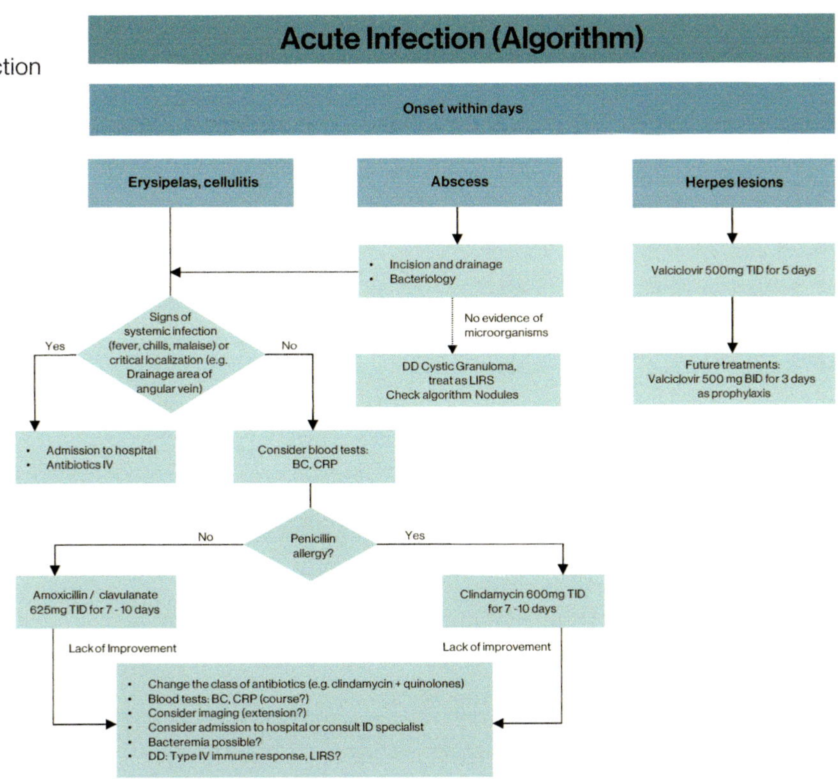

2.3.2 Viral infection

Reactivation of Herpes simplex is the most common viral infection to occur after filler injection. Preferred locations are the lip skin, vermillion border, nasal mucosa, and mucosa of hard palate. Patients with a history of cold sores or fever blisters may be treated prophylactically with valacyclovir 500mg BID for 3 days, specifically when the treatment is targeting the lips or mouth area. If the patient has not received prophylactic treatment, but infection is recognized within 24 hours, valaciclovir at a dose of 500 mg BID for 5 days is recommended (Figure 10).[20,21] Candida species may sometimes cloud the diagnosis and should be kept in consideration, especially in immunocompromised patients and those not responding to treatment with antiviral agents.[46] When blistering is seen beyond the area of the patient's usual area of the herpes simplex virus infection, vascular compromise should be seriously considered (see chapter 2.5 vascular compromise).

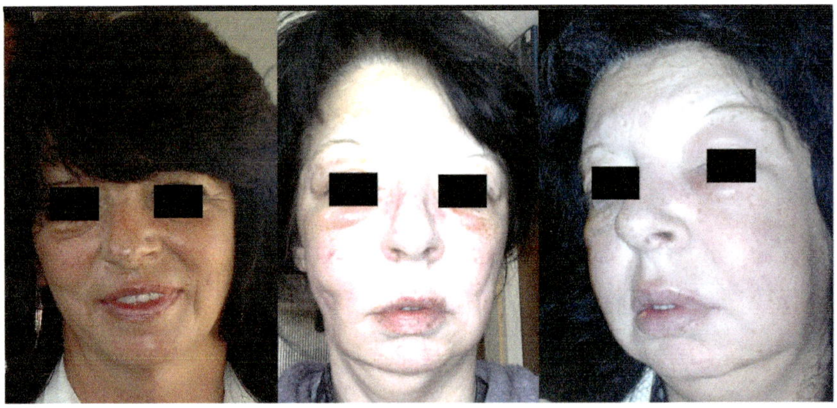

Figure 11
Example of a product-related complication (late inflammatory reaction syndrome, LIRS, discussed in Chapter 2.4) after hyaluronic acid filler injection

From left to right: before - active phase initial presentation - active phase edema, a few days after initial presentation (recurring every 3-4 weeks).

nodules

2.4 Nodules

Nodules are elevated lesions on or in the skin but can also develop in deeper tissues or internal organs, and is a clinical description.[47,48] The clinical finding of a nodule does not indicate anything on the cause, and therefore, it is important to establish the appropriate working diagnosis (Figure 12). Nodules can be caused by incorrect positioning of filler material, overcorrection, accumulation or migration of the product, infection, or as a result from a foreign body reaction.[49,50] Even though the term nodule is often interchanged with granuloma, it is a different entity. Contrary to nodules – which are just a clinal description – granulomas are a histological diagnosis and are typically the result of an overshooting foreign body reaction (see chapter 2.4.3). It is important to distinguish between different types of nodules since they have their own pathological pathway and need a different treatment strategy (Figure 13).

Nodules can be classified by the time of onset (i.e., early and late onset nodules), as well as the type of nodule (i.e., non-inflammatory and inflammatory). In the management of nodules, it is important to determine the right classification, as this will determine the therapy. Below an overview of the recognition and treatment of each class.

Figure 12
Nodules (Differential Diagnosis)

Nodules (Differential Diagnosis)

	Non-inflammatory	Inflammatory	
Diagnosis / type	Accumulated filler material / implant nodule	Biofilm possible → (Genetic factors, Product factors, Immunological factors) →	Chronic granulomatous reaction
		Late Inflammatory Response Syndrome (LIRS)	
Time of occurrence	• Usually immediate • Sometimes delayed occurrence due to migration of the filler material	• After weeks to months, sometimes years	
Pathophysiology	• Accumulated filler: overcorrection, migration • Implant nodule: mild foreign body reaction to the filler is physiological; excessive reaction may lead to a fibrotic, encapsulated implant nodule	• Biofilm seems pivotal by inducing a permanent immune response, thus leading to a chronic granulomatous reaction • Other immunological phenomena may play a role (e.g. excessive foreign body reaction, Type IV reaction, etc.) • Occasionally another infection (e.g. flu, gastroenteritis) may precede and trigger LIRS • Product factors and patient factors play a role	
Clinical presentation	• Painless, non-sore resistance	• Inflammatory, tender nodules	• Inflammatory nodules, plaques or seldom cysts • All areas where the filler is present may react • Histology: Sclerosing, edematous or cystic granuloma • Progression of fibrosis over time
Differential diagnosis	• Deep situated hematoma, encapsulated hematoma • Abscess	• Fluctuating nodule: abscess • Sarcoidosis	
Therapy	• Accumulated filler material: redistribution by massage: after hyaluronidase (HA) or saline/sterile water injection (CaHA) • Encapsulated implant nodule: intra-lesional corticosteroids often not successful, excision may be required	• Consider broad spectrum antibiotics • HA: Hyaluronidase	• HA: Hyaluronidase • Intra-lesional corticosteroids • Intra-lesional 5-FU
Prophylaxis	• Avoid overcorrection	• Creating an aseptic environment during treatments! • Avoiding products that seem to be more prone than others to develop a LIRS	

nodules

Figure 13
Nodules (Algorithm)

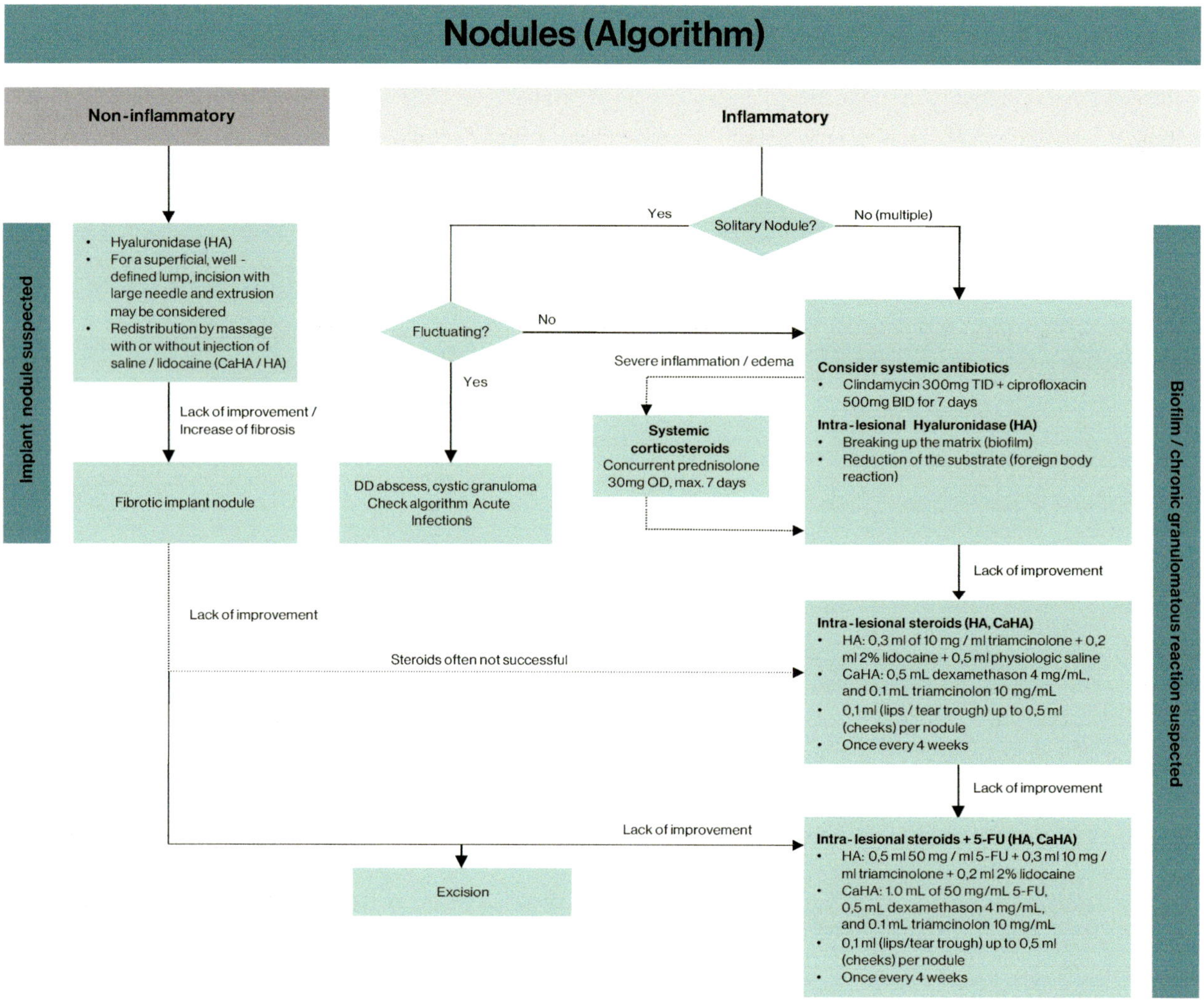

2.4.1 Early onset, non-inflammatory nodules

These type of nodules usually are the result of the injection technique, when excess or inappropriate (e.g., too superficially or incorrect filler selection in dynamic areas) filler placement is applied. These nodules may present directly after injection or after several weeks. Clinically, non-inflammatory nodules are locally confined, hard, well-defined nodules that do not grow in size over time.[21] Overcorrection can be resolved with massaging of the product, and redistributing the product over a larger surface area. If the nodule persists, the treatment is dependent on the product used. If nodules occur after treatment with a HA filler, then injecting hyaluronidase (HYAL) will resolve the nodule. Sometimes a second treatment with HYAL is necessary. Some patients are afraid of dissolving their natural HA, but this is reversible and never a reason not to treat nodules. Besides, native HA has a short half-life of 3 to 5 minutes in the blood, less than a day in the connective tissue and 1 to 3 weeks in the cartilage.[116]
If the non-Inflammatory nodule occurs after injection of a non-HA filler there are less treatment options. CaHA nodules may respond to strong massage or to injection of saline or sterile water (after anesthesia). This will create an osmotic gradient, which aids in the redistribution of the product. It is important to do this within 4-6 weeks. Waiting longer may complicate treatment, because CaHA activates collagen stimulation which forms a strong scaffold around the CaHA micro spheres and will make redistribution more difficult. Early non-inflammatory PLLA nodules may respond to the massage, and saline injection protocol.[51]

2.4.2 Early onset, inflammatory nodules

These type of nodules are usually infection related and have an onset within days to a maximum of two weeks. It should be distinguished from the 'normal' inflammatory reaction of filler injections as the normal reaction needs no treatment. For treatment information, please refer to chapter 2.3.1.

2.4.3 Late onset, non-inflammatory nodules

Late onset non-inflammatory nodules are most often the result of PLLA and particulate fillers (e.g., CaHA). Migration and accumulation of these products leads to this type of nodules. The first step in treatment is to try to disrupt the nodule mechanically by rigorous massaging or needle punctures. If the nodule does not resolve spontaneously, it sometimes can react to intralesional injection of medication. The recommended treatment would be to start with intralesional injection of steroids. Small amounts should be used to prevent skin atrophy. If unsuccessful, a series of intralesional injection of 5-fluorouracil (5-FU), triamcinolone and lidocaine can be considered. The suggested dosage is 0,5 mL of 50 mg/ml 5-FU, 0,3 ml of 10 mg/ml triamcinolone (or 40 mg/ml triamcinolone, depending on localization), and 0,2 mL 2% lidocaine with adrenaline. The amount depends on the localization of the nodule, in a delicate area such as the tear trough or the lips it is obviously less than a nodule deep on the periosteal plane in an area such as the chin. An interesting case report showed that a CaHA nodule resolved > 90% after one week with 0.2 mL injected from a 1.6 mL mix comprised of 1.0 mL of 50 mg/mL 5-FU, 0,5 mL dexamethason 4 mg/mL, and 0.1 mL triamcinolon 10 mg/mL.[144] If a gel carrier from a particulated filler is absorbed and is forming a nodule, there are some reports that a fractionated laser can improve visible material in lips and lower eyelids. As a last resort, excision of injected material that is forming nodules is also an option, but understandably this is only used if all other options failed.

2.4.4 Late onset, inflammatory nodules (late inflammatory response syndrome, LIRS)

Late onset inflammatory nodules are usually the clinical expression of granulomas. The word granuloma comes from the Latin granulum (little grain) and the Greek onkoma (tumor or nodule). It is a inflammatory, granulomatous tissue reaction to, but not exclusively, bacteria or foreign bodies like injectable fillers. It is the ultimate attempt of the body to isolate and get rid of the culprit. To better understand how this could happen after a filler injection, let's first look at the physiological changes that take place after the injection:
Once an HA filler is injected into the tissue, a foreign body reaction will inevitably be initiated as part of the normal, physiological response. Within the first days of injection, neutrophilic granulocytes and monocytes migrate into the area and after about 3 weeks epithelioid cells and aggregated macrophages (foreign body giant cells) are formed, starting phagocytosis of the HA particles. After about 4 weeks, fibroblasts proliferate with increased synthesis and deposition of collagen fibers[54]. This biostimulation contributes positively to the rejuvenation effect of filler treatments and is therefore desirable. However, in rare cases, a physiological foreign body reaction can get out of hand and turn into a pathological, granulomatous inflammatory reaction. Histological examination will then usually show an infiltration with CD4+ T lymphocytes, which secrete cytokines such as IFN-γ, TNF-α, and IL-12, leading to continuous, excessive macrophage activation and inflammation. Histologic distinction can be made between sclerosing, edematous, and cystic granulomas. Clinical findings will most commonly show nodules or plaques; rarely, cystic changes may also occur, and may be confused with an abscess.

Granulomatous inflammatory reactions usually begin no earlier than 3 to 4 weeks after injection but can occur months or even years later. The pathophysiology behind the development of granulomatous inflammation after filler injections is complex and multifactorial. Shape and size of the filler particles play a role in macrophage activation[34] and the fragment size of the degraded hyaluronan chains also appear to exert both activating and suppressive influences on the macrophages[35]. Genetic factors also seem to play a role; for example, implanted fillers may lead to T-cell activation in predisposed patients, probably via Toll-like receptors of the innate immune system[208].

nodules

Certain genetic haplotypes (HLA-B*08 and DRB1*03) seem to be more prone to develop granulomatous inflammatory reactions[188] . Often, a trivial infection (flu-like illness, gastroenteritis) serves as a trigger, whereas the shift in the immune system's reactivity level, e.g., due to altered interferon levels, is likely to be pivotal. This is indicated by the fact that interferon therapies, such as those previously used to treat chronic hepatitis C disease, are able to trigger granulomatous inflammation in areas of filler implants[209].

Interestingly, there are significant differences in the incidence of inflammatory late reactions between different injectors, even when they use the same product. Since the biggest difference between injectors is likely to be how strict they are about sterility, it is reasonable to assume that microbiological factors also play a key role in the development of late inflammatory reactions. Indeed, both Bjarnsholt and Christensen were able to detect bacteria by biopsies of nodules in inflammatory late reactions in virtually all cases, in some cases up to five years after injection[210,211]. The most frequently found culprits were S. epidermidis and P. acnes, i.e., classic inhabitants of the skin microbiome. Furthermore, the bacteria could be found in clusters in each case, which is typical for biofilms. It was demonstrated that HA fillers are an excellent nutrient and growth medium for biofilms. Furthermore, Nygart et al. demonstrated that the use of a single dose of azithromycin in combination with moxifloxacin prior to implantation of a PMMA filler (more on permanent fillers is discussed in chapter 3) could reduce the rate of late inflammatory reactions from 7% to 2% ($p=0.03$; OR 3.7)[212]. Even if the findings from this PMMA filler trial cannot simply be assumed for HA fillers, there seems to be considerable evidence that low-grade infections / biofilms may play a decisive role in the pathogenesis of late inflammatory reactions in HA fillers as well.

In conclusion, we can say that it is the interplay of multiple factors that leads to late onset nodules. As a late inflammatory reaction is always a multifactorial disease, we like to refer to it as a Late Inflammatory Response Syndrome (LIRS). Sometimes it is also referred to as Delayed Onset Nodules (DON). However, even though nodules are a common finding in delayed inflammatory reactions, they are not mandatory. Thus, we prefer the term LIRS. Clinical signs of LIRS are:

- erythema
- edema
- tenderness and
- palpable nodules,
  whereas at least 2 out of 4 signs should be present and symptoms should appear no earlier than 3 weeks after injection

When treating LIRS the first step consists of a few days of watchful waiting before taking any intervention in most cases. The COVID-19 pandemic, bringing along a high number of LIRS cases either by the infection by SARS-CoV-2 itself or by the vaccination against the former (both reactions having different trigger mechanisms, more on the subject can be found in the highlighted box below), showed, that most cases of LIRS resulted in a single, short-lasting bout of an inflammatory reaction with a benign spontaneous course[213]. Therefore a few days of watchful waiting seems to be a reasonable recommendation without putting the patient at unnecessary risk and / or altering the overall prognosis of the disease.

Second, in case of HA the use of hyaluronidase (HYAL) as the first line treatment is recommended, even in cases where a bacterial contamination / biofilm is suspected to play a role in this multifactorial disease. HYAL will help breaking down not only the crosslinked hyaluronic acid but also the matrix of the biofilm embedded within. As the culprits involved in these low-grade infections usually consist of relatively non-virulent bacteria such as *p.acnes*, exposing them is more likely to lead to their clearance through the immune system than to cause a flare up of the infectious process.

Even though the use of antibiotics is suggested in most guidelines (and also still included in our own algorithm), we recommend against the use of antibiotics in most cases. Even if a patient's condition improves on antibiotics, it is not understood whether this is due to the anti-microbial effect of the antibiotic, or rather due to either the anti-inflammatory effect that some of the generally used compounds such as clarithromycin or doxycycline have, or due to the mostly benign natural course of the disease itself. Given that and considering the risk of substantially altering the patient's microbiome with the intervention, we believe that the use of antibiotics in LIRS may not be justified in many cases and thus should be avoided if possible.

Second-line treatment may consist of a series of intralesional injection of triamcinolone, which can be escalated with 5-fluorouracil (5-FU). Artzi et al. recommend the use of a combination of IL triamcinolone (10–20 mg/mL), 5-FU, and saline or lidocaine 1% in a 1:1:1 ratio, whereas Snozzi and Van Loghem[20], Funt and Pavicic[21] recommend using a 3:5:2 ratio (see Figure 13).[142] As with late onset non-inflammatory nodules, the type of nodules may respond to heat (ultrasound, radiofrequency or intralesional laser) aiding in the dissolvement of the nodule.[56] Intralesional heat leads to the liquefaction of the HA microparticles and a mild decrease of bacterial counts on the biofilm. As a last resort, excision of the nodule can be considered. Often inflammatory granulomatous reactions do not have well-defined borders, growing more fingerlike into surrounding tissue, making excision a complicated procedure.

Additional possible treatment options

Recently, immunomodulation with low doses of methotrexate was suggested for the treatment of LIRS.[172] Even though the sample of this case report was low (n=4), low dose methotrexate appeared to offer a low-risk therapeutic alternative in resistant and severe LIRS.

LIRS and vaccinations

After the world-wide start of the COVID-19 vaccinations, reports of vaccine-related LIRS have been published.[173,174] A potential mechanism for LIRS to fillers in COVID-19 related cases is binding and blockade of angiotensin 2 converting enzyme receptors (ACE2), which are targeted by the SARS-CoV-2 virus spike protein to gain entry into the cell. Spike protein interaction with dermal ACE2 receptors favors a pro-inflammatory cascade, promoting a T lymphocyte mediated reaction to granulomas, which formed around residual HA particles. Low dose angiotensin converting enzyme inhibitor (ACE-I, Lisinopril 5-10mg OD) was utilized for treatment, to reduce pro-inflammatory Angiotensin II. ACE inhibitors may therefore have a role in the future for treatment of LIRS. More research is required to evaluate the potential of ACE-I as potential additions to our LIRS algorithms.

If a patient develops LIRS after a vaccination (e.g. COVID-19), corticosteroids should be avoided because it will compromise the effect of the vaccine. It is common sense to postpone any vaccinations (including travel vaccinations) as long as a patient is under corticosteroid medication.

2.5 Prevention and management of vascular complications

Vascular complications are considered as one of the most severe, yet rare, complications following treatment with STF and require immediate and adequate medical treatment. Depending on the extent of the intravascular embolus, the clinical effect can range from asymptomatic to devastating and life changing. Embolization of the central retinal artery may lead to irreversible blindness. While the incidence of vascular compromise remains low, more cases are appearing, mainly due to the increased use of STF and more advanced indications being performed by a greater number of practitioners worldwide.[59-61] Two main types of ischemia are discussed in this chapter: peripheral ischemia (potentially leading to tissue necrosis and scarring) and central (retinal) ischemia (potentially leading to blindness).[5,6]

Vascular compromise is the disruption of blood supply to an artery or vein. It can happen in any area of the face (or body), but this chapter only focuses on the face. When the injector causes peripheral ischemia, a sudden onset of blanching, followed by livedo reticularis and/or blue-grayish discoloration will occur. In central ischemia, the embolus may displace proximally to cerebral arteries via the ophthalmic artery, leading to neurological symptoms like aphasia or even hemiparesis. Vascular compromise of branches of the ophthalmic artery could lead to a sudden onset of simultaneous occurrence of vision loss (e.g. occlusion of the central retinal artery), eye pain, ophthalmoparesis and eyelid ptosis.. Ophthalmoparesis, ptosis, vertigo and fainting may occur simultaneously, as well as the abovementioned peripheral ischemic symptoms.[62,73] It is critical to recognize these complications as soon as possible so that treatment can be started immediately. While there are several hours of time to restore peripheral circulation before necrosis will commence, there may be only a very short window of opportunity as short as 15 minutes to restore retinal circulation, before blindness becomes irreversible. [5,6,68,202]
Vascular compromise to the retina can result in permanent blindness if the central retinal artery is occluded. Due to the short distance to the central retinal artery, injections of STF in the glabellar region are most likely to cause retinal occlusion.[76]

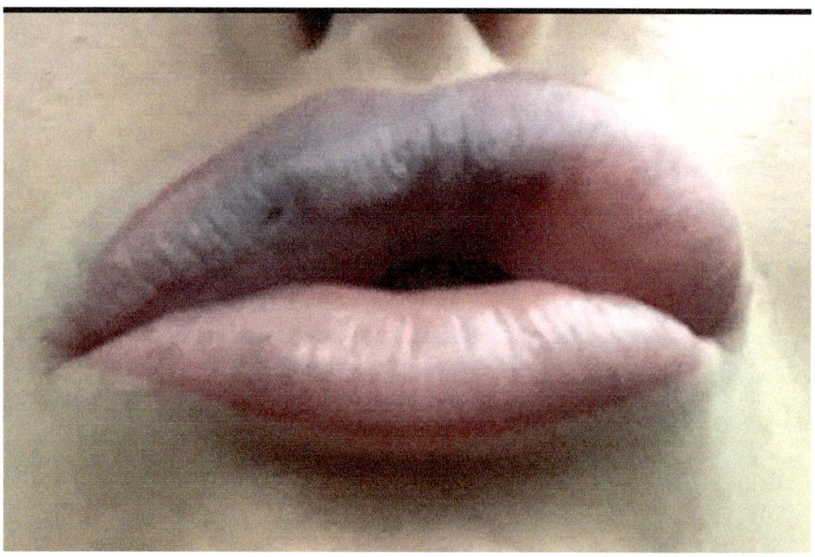

Figure 14
Lip ischemia

Embolization of the superior labial artery.
Note the similarity with a hematoma.
Image courtesy Tom Decates, MD PhD.

Direct arterial embolization may occur in an anterograde (with the blood stream) or retrograde (against the bloodstream) fashion. Anterograde vascular occlusion causes a decreased blood flow downstream to the vascular branches, resulting in visible surface changes of the skin.[6] Retrograde vascular occlusion allows the STF to travel against the arterial blood flow. The product often travels back to a vascular bifurcation and the embolus can then subsequently cause anterograde occlusion at a more proximal or distal location than the initial injection site.[6]

The arterial occlusion results in reduction of arterial perfusion, which was most noted to occur within the distal capillaries, as demonstrated in a mouse animal model.[75] Apart from arterial embolization, venous embolization is a possible cause of vascular occlusion.

However, as veins increase in diameter downstream of the capillary bed, arterial occlusion seems more relevant. Venous compression is a theoretical possibility for outflow obstruction from the capillary bed, also causing stasis of capillary perfusion, but as evidence for this possible pathogenetic pathway is absent, we will only focus on arterial embolization. Besides mechanical obstruction, two other factors may play an essential role in causing hypoperfusion after HA is injected intravascularly: First, the highly irritant effect of HA on vessel walls leading to inflammation and coagulation, and second, choke vessel closure between angiosomes (see section on choke vessels on Page 19).

A thorough understanding of peripheral arterial anatomy is essential in order to reduce the risk of both retinal and peripheral ischemia. General statements can be made concerning the expected anatomical layer and the general direction of the arteries (Table 2). Injection techniques can be adjusted in order to reduce the risk of vascular complications. Large boluses should be avoided.[62,73] Positioning the bevel of the needle or cannula in a different anatomical layer to that where the artery is most likely to be found, and injecting perpendicular to the expected direction of an artery, can also reduce the risk of injecting large amounts intravascularly.[5,6] A detailed anatomy of the facial vasculature is described elsewhere.[74]

In a large global review of blindness secondary to facial filler injections, Beleznay et al. reported a total of 146 cases, although this inevitably represents underreporting.[76,77] The most common locations for filler injections causing vision changes were the nasal region (n = 52), the glabella (n = 51), the forehead (n = 21), and the nasolabial fold (NLF) (n = 20).[76,77] Less common sites were the temple, cheek, chin, and upper eyelid.[77] Historically, autologous fat injections caused the most visual compromise complications, attributed to the larger volumes and needle bore size necessary. However, for the years 2015 to 2018, 81.3% of visual impairment/loss caused by STF occurred with the injection of a hyaluronic acid. This reflects the increase in popularity of hyaluronic acid during this period.[77]

In particular, the supratrochlear artery, which is itself a terminal branch of the ophthalmic artery, can be inadvertently accessed due to its superomedial location at the orbit and its extensive vascular anastomoses throughout the forehead and with the adjacent supraorbital artery.[6]

Embolization of the posterior ciliary arteries, which provide a blood supply to the optic nerve, may cause optic neuropathy. Lastly, occlusion of the middle cerebral artery, a branch of the internal carotid artery, can occur with significant injection pressure and result in cerebral infarction.[77]

Although the risks of STF-associated vascular compromise cannot be eliminated completely, there are multiple steps a physician can take to avoid such complications. First of all, the patient must be well informed about the risks of the treatment, and informed consent must be obtained before any procedure begins. Physicians are also advised to assemble an "emergency tool kit" for the management of complications should they arise.[17] During the treatment, there are several recommendations to further reduce the risk of vascular filler complications; the ten most important are listed in chapter 1.4. In the appendix, chapter 5 of this book, we have listed our UMA filler first aid that we believe should be present whenever performing STF treatments.

Recently, reports have been published promoting the use of doppler ultrasound (DUS) scans prior to injection of STF.[82] The rationale is that due to high arterial anatomic variations, the exact location of arteries remains unknown until they can actually be visualized. This technique may allow large diameter arteries to be localized. Caution should be taken when using DUS during injection as a difference of 1 mm could mean the difference between intra- and extra-arterial injection. However, DUS can be useful with large bolus injection with the gunshot technique (e.g., fossa temporalis).

vascular complications

Whereas the use of Doppler Ultrasound (DUS) has several advantages after proper training and experience, there are some disadvantages associated with the use of DUS as a preventative tool for the avoidance of intravascular injection[5,6]:

The injector may have a false sense of security: the smaller diameter arteries cannot be seen due to the limited resolution of most devices. As we have learnt from cadaver dissections with dye-colored arteries, the facial tissues are supplied by thousands of smaller diameter arteries that interconnect with the arterial system. Delorenzi compared the arterial network to 'an interstate highway system, where even the smallest dirt roads eventually connect to the interstate highway and the driver can reach any destination'.[66] Similarly, in the face, injecting in a smaller diameter artery, invisible on the US screen, can lead to wide-spread necrosis, just as injecting in larger arteries can.

Smaller needles cannot be used as injection under visualization is virtually impossible with thin and short needles. The thinner needles (27-30G, 13 mm) that are generally used for HA injection are difficult to see under US. Even more importantly, these needles are usually introduced perpendicular to the skin, which is not an ideal angle for US visualization. If the needles enter at a smaller angle to the skin, their short length makes deep injections impossible.

The non-dominant hand is unavailable for guiding the injection. Many expert injectors agree that the non-dominant hand is at least as important as the injecting hand. Often, the non-dominant hand is essential to advance the cannula or needle to a certain target area. Therefore, the use of DUS-guided injections may reduce the aesthetic outcome of STF treatments.

There are sterility issues: the injector has to use sterile US gel and a sterile protective rubber condom around the probe, as well as ensure that the gel itself does not enter the skin though the needle holes.

The main advantage of DUS as a preventative measure is that the injector can form a general idea of the location of the arteries. It is important that injectors using DUS preventatively are aware of the limited sensitivity of this safety test and practice the suggested technical preventative measures mentioned in chapter 1. More information on DUS imaging in filler complication can be found in chapter 4.4.

Four different types of arterial occlusion will be discussed: peripheral and central (retinal) ischemia after dermal filler injection with HA or CaHA. It is important to realize that any particulate or viscous gel can lead to vascular compromise. For example, poly-L-lactic acid (PLLA, Sculptra) is a thin, watery suspension when reconstituted, but case reports have been published on vascular compromise after PLLA injection.[83] Since PLLA has no way to reverse or dissolve, the necessary precautions should be taken into account.

2.5.1 Management of peripheral vascular complications after HA injection

When a HA embolism obstructs blood flow, this can potentially lead to tissue anoxia, ischemia and progression to necrosis. The filler material can migrate both antegrade and retrograde along the arterial network. When skin color changes (white, marbling, blue-grey) are observed, suspicion of vascular compromise should increase. An immediate onset of blanching followed by marbling (livedo reticularis) usually occurs within hours after injection due to lack of oxygen resulting in venous dilation. After the livedo reticularis phase, the blue-gray phase follows due to sustained lack of oxygen. Finally, 1–2 days later, the blister (pimple) phase indicates the first signs of skin necrosis. Rapid recognition and treatment of a vascular event is important to avoid serious, potentially life-changing complications (Figure 15 , Video 1, Figures 16 and 17).

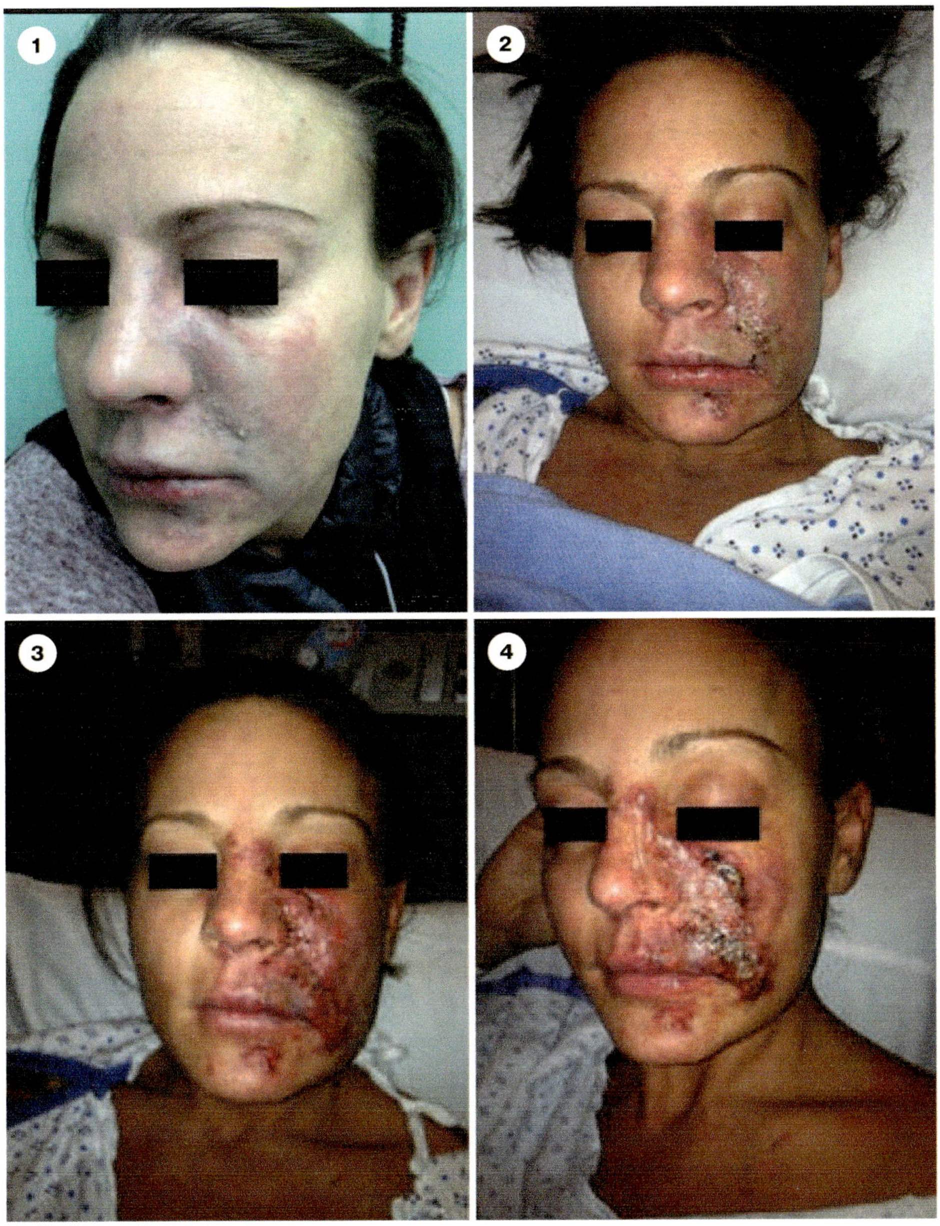

Figure 15
Progression of vascular compromise after an embolic event

From Funt D, Pavicic T, Dermal fillers in aesthetics: an overview of adverse events and treatment approaches, Clinical, Cosmetic and Investigational Dermatology 2013:6 295–316. Originally published by and used with permission from Dove Medical Press Ltd.

Treatment for peripheral ischemia is prompt administration of high-dose hyaluronidase and massage with warm compresses, as well as aspirin to avoid blood coagulation around the HA embolus.[5,6,17,20,30,63-66] A minimum dose of 200 U of hyaluronidase is required, but doses of up to 1500 U have been suggested in the literature.[17] We suggest injecting 500U of hyaluronidase reconstituted in 1ml 2% lidocaine per 5x5 cm of visibly affected skin, injected hourly until capillary refill normalizes (see algorithm in Figure 18) The half-life of hyaluronidase is short, so injections should be repeated at hourly intervals until capillary refill normalizes and tissue necrosis is avoided.[67] The patient should be followed up after 7 days with good progression, or earlier if needed, and after 4 weeks. When infections arise due to the vascular infarction, antibiotic treatment should be started immediately. Reconstitution of hyaluronidase is normally done with saline, but reconstitution with lidocaine without epinephrine may promote vasodilation. Further therapeutic options, even though they have a low evidence level, include low-molecular-weight heparin, pentoxyfillin and hyperbaric oxygen therapy. Figures 18 and 19 show the differential diagnosis and treatment algorithm of vascular complications following HA injections.[6]

With proper training vascular obstructions can be located with a relatively simple and affordable DUS device. The slow flow doppler settings show a clear difference from the normal pulsating arterial image (generally either blue or red colored). However, when there is a vascular obstruction, flow oscillates back and forth, resulting in both blue and red areas inside a vessel; a hypoechoic (black) deposition (of HA) is usually seen downstream of the chaotic flow area. With proper training, an aesthetic practitioner can learn to perform DUS-guided intravascular hyaluronidase injections. DUS guided hyaluronidase injections allow restoration of flow with minimal dosage compared to the standard protocol.[82] Clinically, the skin will show immediate signs of reperfusion after dissolving the embolus (pink reactive hyperemia).

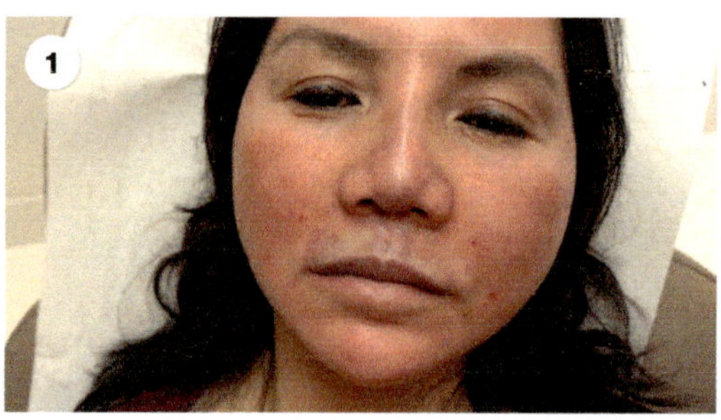

30 minutes after treatment

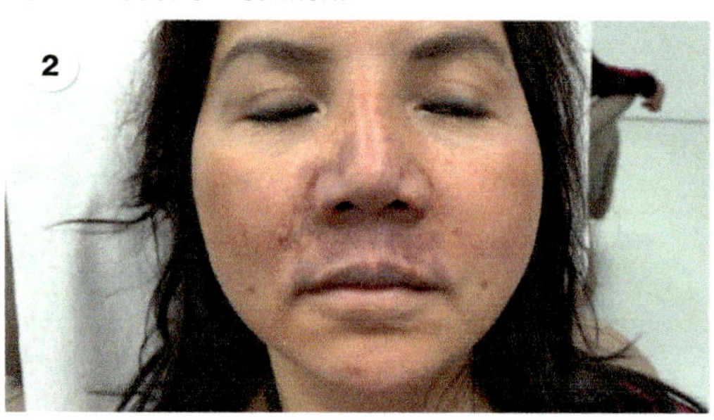

1 day after treatment

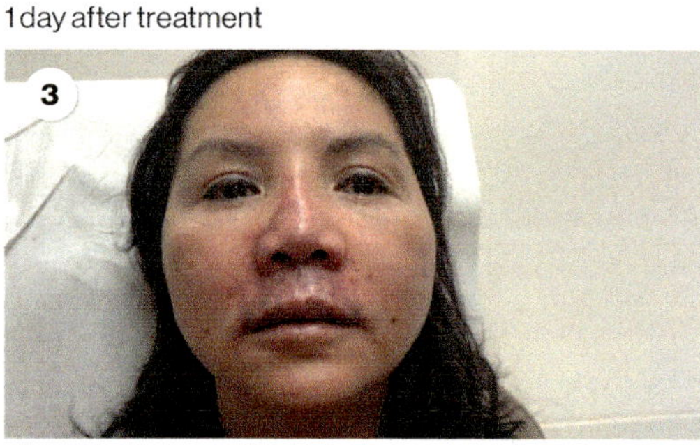

2 days after treatment

Watch videos at http://bit.ly/Complication-Prevention-and-Management

Video 1

Example of peripheral vascular event after HA injection in the columella with ischemic symptoms in the nose and lip

First video is 30 minutes after HA treatment, note blanching and livedo reticularis symptoms without pain. The second video is one day later, the third video is two days after treatment.

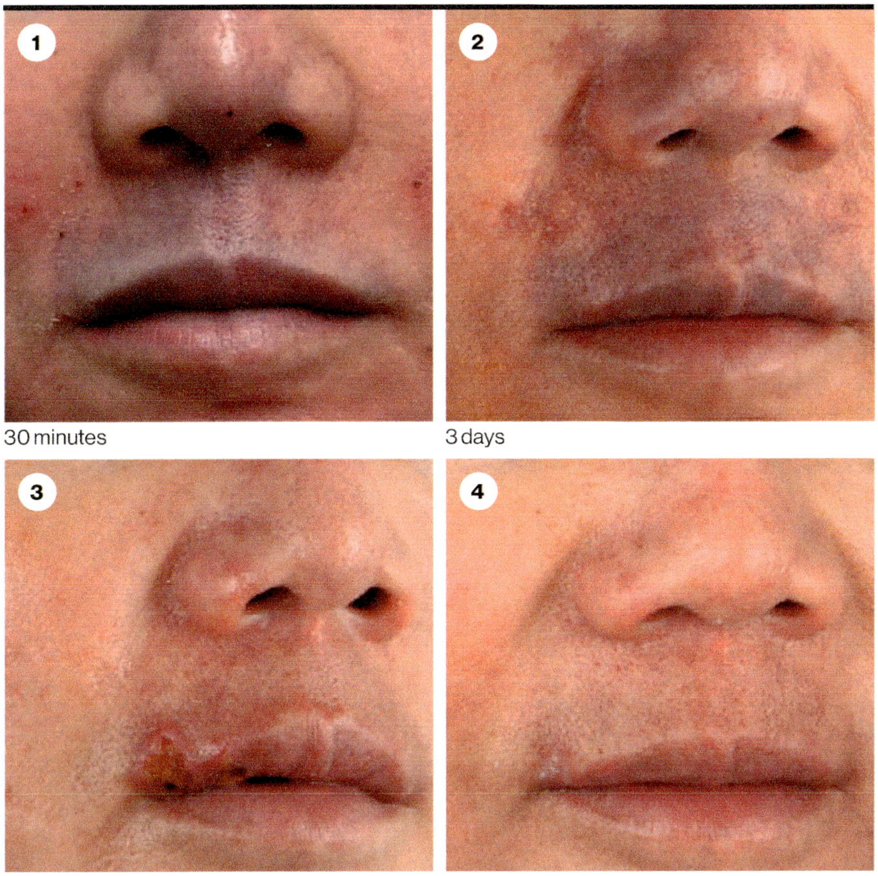

30 minutes | 3 days | 12 days | 23 days

Figure 16
This is the same patient as in the above video. Different stages after HA injection in the columellar artery with ischemia in the nose and upper lip. The patient was treated with the previous more conservative protocol including hyaluronidase (3x 150U), tadalafil, aspirin, warm compresses, PRP, and hyperbaric oxygen.

Note the open wound in Figure 16.3. on day 12.

vascular complications

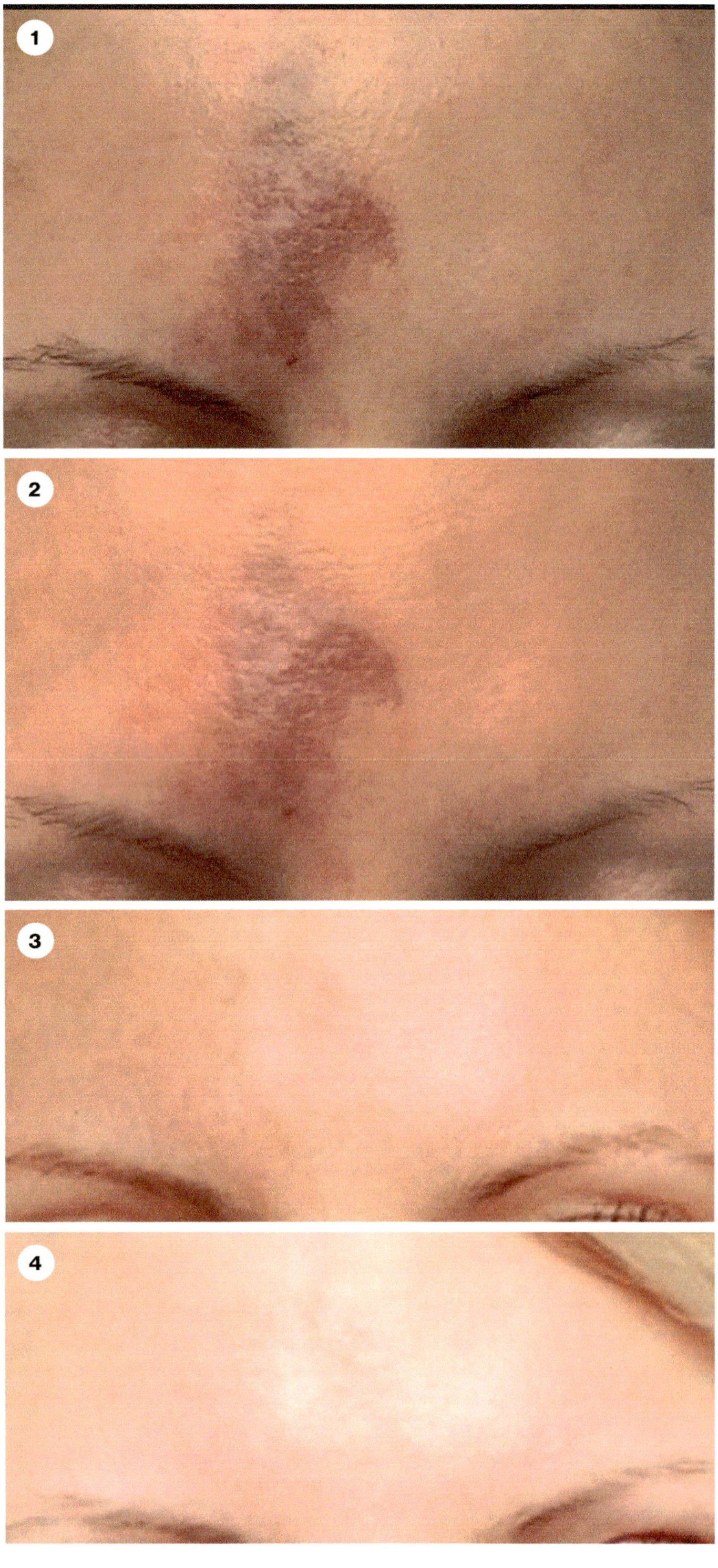

Figure 17

Peripheral vascular event after HA in the supratrochlear artery. The high dose pulsed protocol was used starting 4 days after treatment (patient delay).

1 four days after treatment (3x 1000U)
2 six days after treatment (daily 3x 1000U)
3 one month after treatment
4 two months after treatment.

Note: no wound arose despite the late start of treatment.

2.5.2 Management of retinal ischemia after HA injections

Due to the potential severity of vascular complications, the authors strongly recommend that all injectors should receive special training in the theoretical background and practical skill set of complication management, given that (immediate) referral to an ophthalmologist may be too late as the time frame to restore reperfusion to the ischemic retina may be as short as 15 minutes.[202] When a patient complains of immediate visual loss, blurring and potential central nervous system symptoms as vertigo, unconsciousness and nausea, retinal ischemia should be suspected, and immediate action is required. Treatment recommendations still have a low level of evidence as they are primarily based on expert opinions. A single drop of topical timolol 0.5% can be applied to the affected eye to reduce the intraocular pressure.[20,68] Rebreathing air in a (paper) bag may increase CO_2 concentration and thereby reduce intraocular pressure further.[20,68] Carruthers et al. have suggested retrobulbar injections of hyaluronidase in case of HA injection.[69,70]
Ophthalmologists recommend injecting hyaluronidase in the retrobulbar space only when the patient has no light perception (NLP) or when the patient sees no hand movement. If the patient can still count fingers, no retrobubulbar injection is advised (see text box on retrobulbar hyaluronidase injection and ocular massage). Differential diagnosis of acute visual loss, although very unlikely, include migraine aura and a stroke unrelated to the injection.

After injection of hyaluronidase and during transportation to the hospital, ocular massage should be continued in an attempt to push the embolus through the retinal capillary vessels into the venous system and to reduce intra ocular pressure. Other therapies to improve retinal perfusion described in the literature (albeit with limited success) may be considered and include immediate, hyperbaric therapy/oxygen, diuretics, systemic and topical corticosteroids, anticoagulation, and needle decompression of the anterior chamber.[78] In the hospital, additional therapies may be considered (Figure 18).[5,6]

Figure 18
Peripheral ischemia after HA or CaHA according to Van Loghem JAJ, Siebenga P and Thuis J.[5]

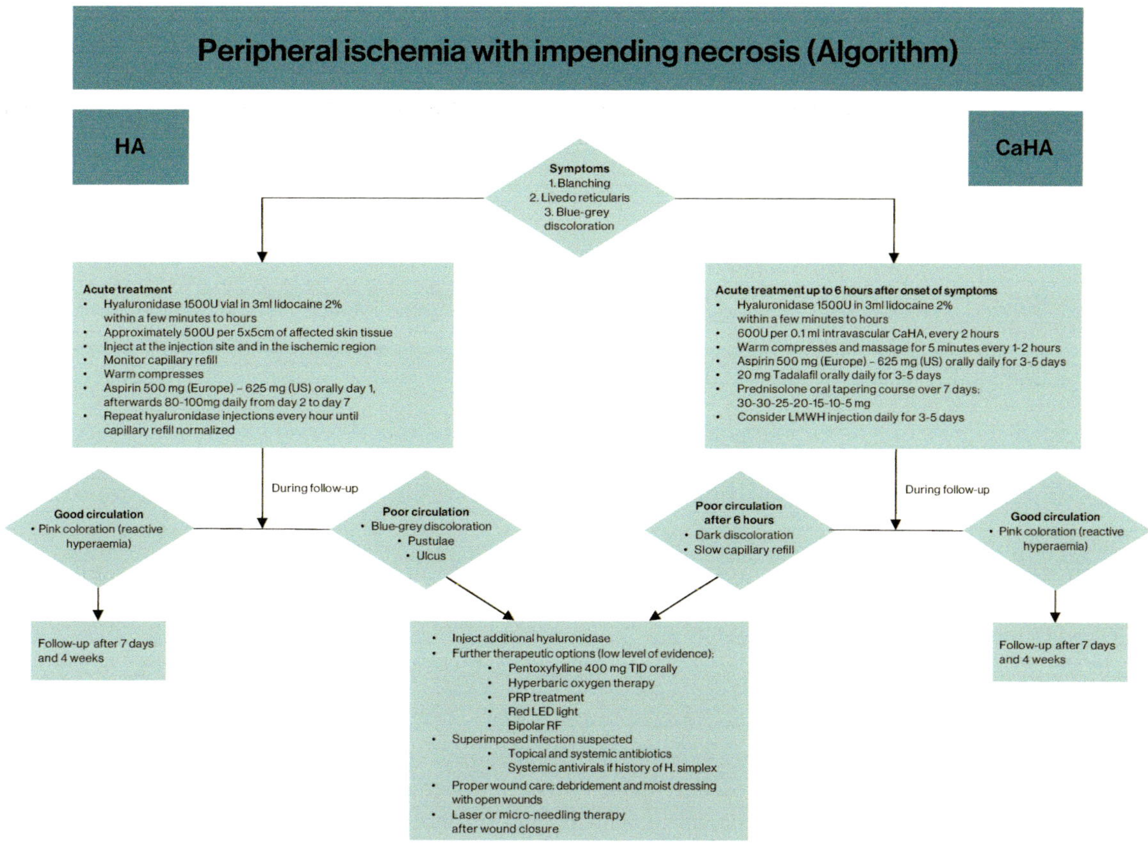

vascular complications

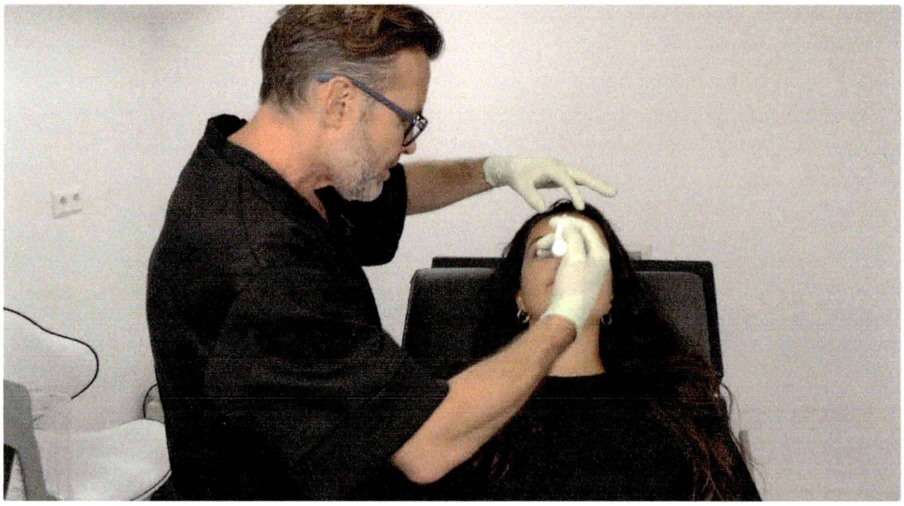

Watch video at http://bit.ly/Complication-Prevention-and-Management

Video 2
Simulation of management of acute visual loss after HA injection

Figure 19
Acute Blindness after HA or CaHA according to Van Loghem JAJ, Siebenga P and Thuis, J [5]

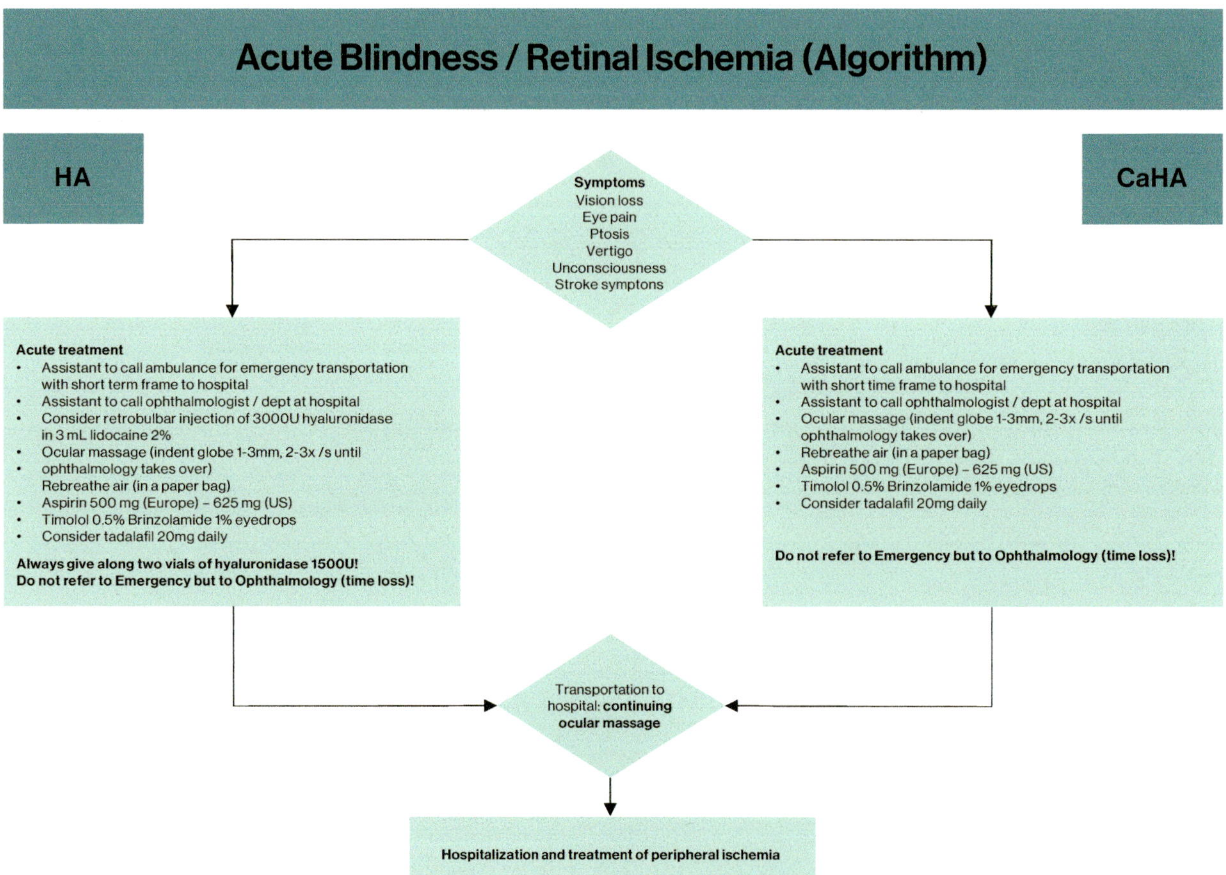

Retrobulbar injection

Retrobulbar injection with hyaluronidase is widely known as a potentially sight-saving treatment after STF-induced blindness. However, the use of it is still controversial, as there is insufficient evidence that either supports or advises against retrobulbar injections.

The main problem is the lack of evidence that retrobulbar injection with hyaluronidase is effective. There are few case reports in the literature showing improvement in visual acuity after retrobulbar injection of hyaluronidase. The few cases with a positive outcome that exist, either have inconsistencies in the report or the visual impairment was due to central retinal artery branch occlusion (BRAO), rather than central retinal artery occlusion (CRAO).[194,195] In all case reports of a true CRAO, no improvement in visual acuity was reported after retrobulbar injection of hyaluronidase.[79,196,197] This is (partly) due to a lack of penetration of hyaluronidase to the dura of the optic nerve[198] in the human eye. Next to that, the efficacy of retrobulbar injections has only been demonstrated in a rabbit model.[199] Since the rabbit retina is merangiotic[200], the clinical relevance to humans seems limited.[201] In rabbits, the central retinal artery supplies only two horizontal bands of the retina.[201] In addition, recent data suggests that retinal infarction is most likely occurs as early as 12-15 minutes after a complete CRAO, as opposed to the previously assumed 90-240 minutes.[202] Lastly, retrobulbar injections themselves carry risks such as retrobulbar hemorrhage, ocular globe injury, optic nerve damage, and extraocular muscle injury.[203]

The technique for retrobulbar injection must be accurate. The retrobulbar space lies within the extraocular muscle cone, posterior to globe.[204] The entry point of the needle is at the junction between the middle and outer thirds of the inferior orbital rim. Pass the needle just 15 mm below the eye with the bevel facing upward.[204] The needle should be parallel to the floor of the orbit and angled downward.[204] You may feel the resistance from the orbital septum as you push through it. Point the tip of the needle upward and inward toward the top of the skull. As you pierce through the muscle cone, you should feel its resistance.[204]
Not many aesthetic physicians are experienced with this procedure and execute it in a way that is beneficial to the patient. Also, not many ophthalmologists have performed this procedure, except for retinologists. Most of them may be hesitant to deal with this type of situation. One solution to this problem could be to make arrangements in advance with an ophthalmologist in case of emergency.

Despite all these arguments against retrobulbar injection we cannot conclude that it is ineffective since the benefits may outweigh the risks of the procedure in the catastrophic event of complete loss of vision. If the treating practitioner has experience with retrobulbar injections, this could potentially be a crucial step in reducing injury.

2.5.3 Management of peripheral vascular complications after CaHA injection.

Calcium hydroxylapatite (CaHA, Radiesse, Merz Aesthetics GmbH, Frankfurt, Germany) is the most commonly used non-HA filler on the market today.[1,71] HA can induce severe choke reactions, leading to wide spread necrosis, whereas the role of intravascular CaHA in causing choke reactions is less clear. Compared with HA, CaHA has a different clinical presentation of ischemia after intravascular injection and generally more volume is necessary to induce ischemia. CaHA is also usually more forgiving as the product can be distributed and diluted over a larger vascular network without leading to acute ischemia and tissue necrosis. On the other hand, even though most intravascular injections probably remain subclinical with small injection amounts, larger volumes of intravascular CaHA can potentially lead to wide-spread necrosis. Minimizing the amount of injected product is therefore the most important preventative safety measure.[62] After inadvertent intravascular CaHA injection, and in the absence of a reversing agent similar to hyaluronidase for HA fillers, massage and aspirin to prevent clotting are the most important elements of the algorithm (Figure 18).[62]

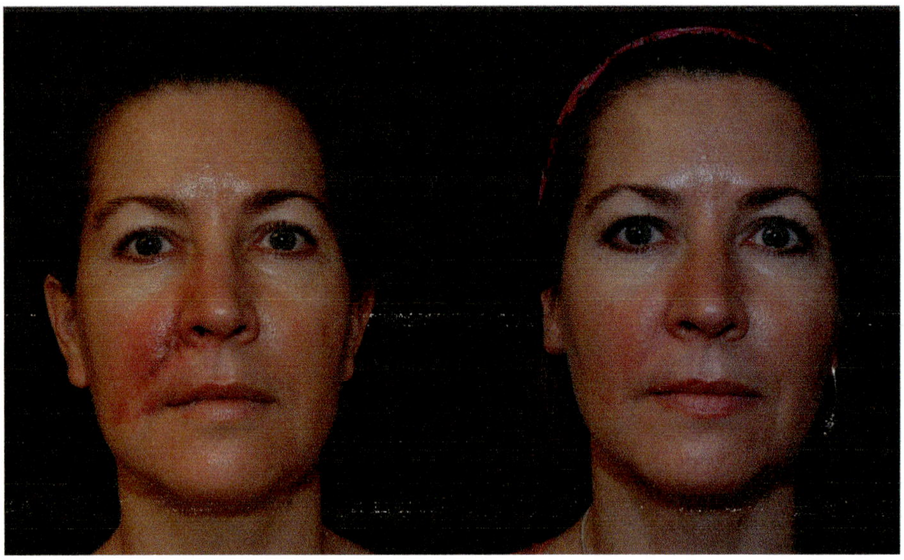

Figure 20
Vascular adverse event due to injection of CaHA in the facial artery

Note complete resolution without permanent skin damage.
Images courtesy David Funt, MD

A CaHA induced vascular adverse event has the same clinical signs appear as with HA embolization: blanching and livedo reticularis. Pain is not always present as the product is generally either mixed with lidocaine or contains lidocaine. The injector generally has an idea of the amount of CaHA that was injected intravascularly. Per 0.1 mL intravascularly injected CaHA, 600U of hyaluronidase reconstituted in lidocaine 2% (without epinephrine) should be injected every 2 hours. The affected area should be injected with hyaluronidase regardless of the filler type due to its edema-reducing and anti-inflammatory properties.[62] Oral aspirin should be administered to prevent upstream clotting and warm massages should be given to increase vasodilation for 5 minutes every 1-2 hours. During the massage, the capillary refill should be noted and the acute treatment should be continued until the capillary refill normalizes to approximately 2s. To further promote vasodilation, tadalafil 20mg can be prescribed and to prevent further clotting over the next days, either low dose aspirin (80-100 mg) and / or low molecular weight heparin (LMWH) can be prescribed. In order to reduce inflammation and tissue pressure due to edema, oral corticosteroids (prednisolone tapering course) can be prescribed. When the patient is known to have herpes simplex virus in the affected area, antiviral treatment is recommended (Valaciclovir 500mg BID for 7 days). If the capillary refill normalizes, follow-up should be planned after 7 days or earlier if necessary. After 4 weeks the final follow-up should be scheduled. If the capillary refill does not normalize completely, additional treatment options include Pentoxyfilline 400 mg TID to increase arterial perfusion, hyperbaric oxygen therapy (HBOT) to increase tissue oxygenation and platelet-rich plasma (PRP) injections to promote angiogenesis and wound healing. Lastly, if an open wound would start to arise, the treating physician should be aware of the possibility that the wound may be extra susceptible to infection due to the fact that the tissue perfusion is reduced by the occlusion. To prevent infections, topical antibiotics should be prescribed and systemic antibiotics can be considered.

2.5.4 Management of retinal ischemia after CaHA injections

As CaHA has no reversing agent, no retrobulbar injection is required. However, there are a few important steps to take in the event of acute visual loss after CaHA injection. The goal is rapid reduction of intraocular pressure to allow the emboli to dislodge downstream and improve retinal perfusion. Acute management involves ocular massage to lower the intraocular pressure and to push the CaHA particles through the retinal vessels to the venous circulation. The technique involves small rapid changes of intraocular pressure over a period of 1-3 hours, until all retinal emboli have been cleared from the vessels. Ocular massage is performed with the patient in a supine position, looking downward with their eyes closed.[5,6,79] Gentle pressure is applied to the sclera of the eye with a finger, indenting the globe by a few millimeters at a frequency of 2-3 times per second.[62,79,80] The prolonged, rapid small changes in intraocular pressure may dislodge the embolus (Video 4). The procedure should be continued until the patient has been transferred to the hospital and is under the care of an ophthalmologist. Carbon dioxide inhalation is another method of vasodilating the retinal arteries to increase the chance of the embolus dislodging and moving downstream.[62,79,81] Additional treatments may include administration of timolol 0.5% eye drops, or other beta-adrenergic antagonists such as brinzolamide or azetazolamide, or oral pentoxifylline, which will reduce intraocular pressure and improve retinal flow, respectively.[62]

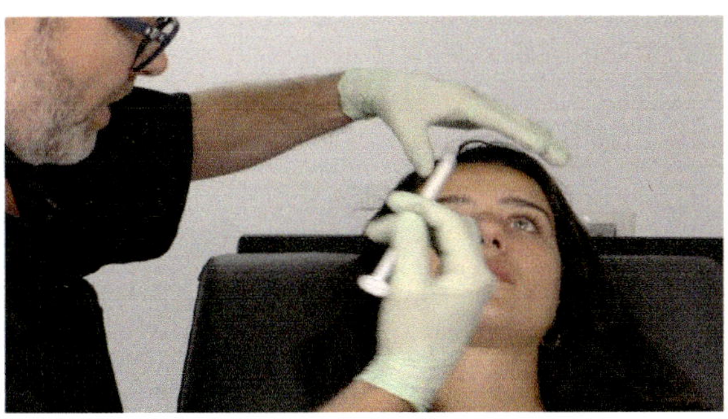

Watch video at http://bit.ly/Complication-Prevention-and-Management

Video 3
Simulation of management of acute visual loss after CaHA injection

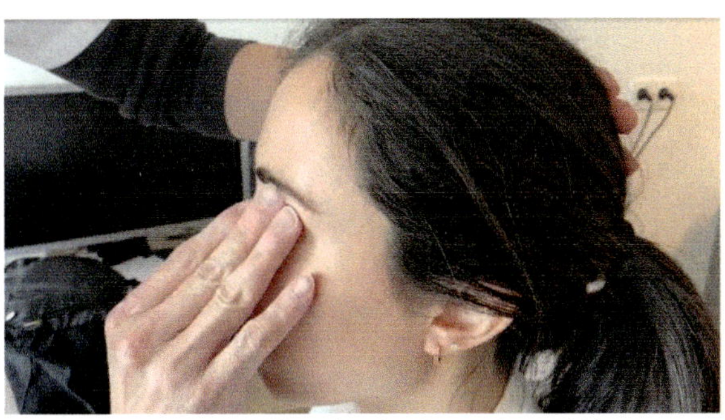

Watch video at http://bit.ly/Complication-Prevention-and-Management

Video 4
Ocular Massage

The latest consensus meeting of ophthalmologists in the Amsterdam University Medical Center resulted in this instructional video. Courtesy prof. Peerooz Saeed, Amsterdam University Medical Center

poly-l-lactic acid complications

2.6 Poly-L-lactic acid (PLLA) complications

PLLA is a biostimulatory product that is placed in the subdermal or periosteal layer and acts via a foreign body reaction; monocyte and leucocyte exsudation, formation of multi-nucleated giant cells around the PLLA particles and a release of cytokines will result in Fibroblast migration that will gradually start producing collagen after three weeks. The PLLA particles will dissolve due to hydrolysis, and the collagen effects will last up to 25 months.[185,186] This section will discuss complications that may occur using the PLLA product commercially marketed as Sculptra®, as the authors (RF, FT) have extensive (>20 years) experience with its use. Sculptra® PLLA particles of approximately 50 micrometres are irregular in surface, and 150 mg is packaged in a vial with mannitol and carboxy methyl cellulose (CMC). Newer products on the market include Lanluma® V and Lanluma® X, which are outside the scope of this section.

This section will focus on a PLLA-specific complication, fibrosis. For other complications, the authors refer to previous recommendations.

2.6.1 Prevention

Knowledge of the product and techniques is necessary, as well as expertise to handle PLLA complications, should they occur. Aspiration prior to injection is a reliable safety test in contrast to more viscous and elastic gels like HA or CaHA products, as PLLA is essentially a watery liquid and, therefore, can be easily aspirated out of the needle lumen. Routinely aspirating prior to injection is advised in order to avoid intravascular injection. The prevalence of PLLA complications has significantly reduced since the 2014 consensus, where the reconstitution volume was increased to 7-10 ml per vial of Sculptra.[147]

PLLA should not be injected in the following anatomical areas

- the peri-orbital area (risk of nodule formation and vascular complications)
- the lips (risk of nodule formation)
- hyperkinetic areas (risk of nodule formation)
- the forehead (risk of vascular complications)

Contra-indications for PLLA use

- Active inflammation or infection in or near the treatment area
- Hypersensitivity to any of the components
- Pregnancy
- Breastfeeding
- Autoimmune diseases
- Interferon therapy

Reconstitution protocol of Sculptra®

01 Sculptra® (1 vial of 150 mg PLLA)

02 Add 5 ml sterile water and shake vigorously 1 minute until a homogeneous suspension

03 Add additional 3 ml of sterile water and shake again until suspension is homogeneous

04 Add lidocaine (1 mL 2%, with or without adrenalin)

05 Shake vigorously

06 Do not inject the foam present on the surface of the PLLA suspension. When shaken a small layer of foam can appear on the surface of the suspension this consists of air and not entirely hydrated parts of PLLA, which when injected can cause nodules.

07 Sculptra® can be used immediately, ore stored for up to 72 hours at room temperaturere

Reconstitution protocols for Lanluma®

01 Lanluma® V: 1 vial + 15 ml sterile water

02 Lanluma® X: 1 vial + 40 ml sterile water

03 Shake vigorously

04 Do not inject foam on top of the suspension in the vial

poly-l-lactic acid complications

2.6.2 PLLA Complications

Non-inflammatory PLLA Nodules

Non-inflammatory nodules can arise depending on the techniques used as well as the facial area where PLLA was injected. They can appear 1-2 months after injection and usually present as a solitary nodule varying from very small, only minimally palpable, to approximately the size of a pea. It is well-defined and confined in a fibrous capsula. The nodule will remain until the PLLA has been resorbed or until it is successfully treated. Histologically, a foreign body reaction is seen where PLLA particles aggregate.

Causes of non-inflammatory PLLA nodules are generally technique dependent

- Too high PLLA concentration due to too little reconstitution volume (<9 ml)
- Too much product injected at a specific site
- Too short interval between PLLA injection sessions <5 weeks
- Inappropriate post-injection distribution by manual massage
- Too superficial (intradermal) injection

Treatment of non-inflammatory PLLA nodules

Direct and firm massage can reduce the nodule. When there is not enough improvement, puncturing the nodule with a needle in order to fragment it can help, especially when followed by an injection of saline (or lidocaine) and a firm massage. This way, the PLLA fragments can be redistributed over a larger surface area and exposed to water so that the PLLA will disperse and the palpable particles will decrease in size.

> Correct reconstitution and application of the product is paramount to avoid PLLA complications.

Late PLLA complications

Granuloma formation after PLLA injection usually presents as several nodules 6-24 months after injection at the areas where PLLA was injected. These late inflammatory nodules are less well defined compared to PLLA nodules and if untreated will remain active for 1-5 years. In the experience of the author (FT), Fitzpatrick type 1 skinned patients as well as patients who have received permanent soft tissue fillers in the past, have most risk of developing granulomas. Histologically, a PLLA induced granuloma is characterized by multi nucleated giant cells, macrophages and lymphocytic infiltration around the PLLA particles.

PLLA granuloma treatment has been well described by Lemperle and Gaulthier-Hazan and is recommended here as well.[146] Treatment options include

- Triamcinolon 20-40 mg intralesionally
- Triamcinolon (10 mg/ml) + 5-fluorouracil (50 mg/ml) intralesionally
- Prednisolon 20-40 mg orally for maximum 1 week
- Betamethason 5-7 mg intralesionally
- 1:3 Betamethason 3,5 mg + 1:3 5-fluorouracil (1,6ml) + 1:3 lidocaine intralesionally

poly-l-lactic acid complications

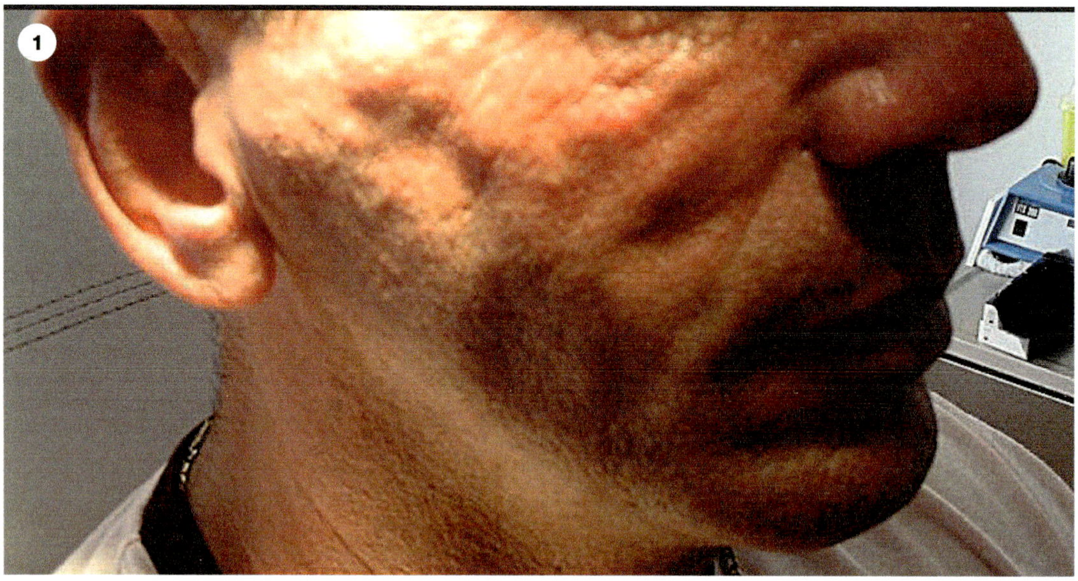

Figure 21.1
Clinical presentation of LIRS (most probably a granuloma)

Note erythematous nodules on the zygoma (3x) and an elongated nodule at the tear trough area. This picture was taken using grazing light in order to visualize the skin elevations better.

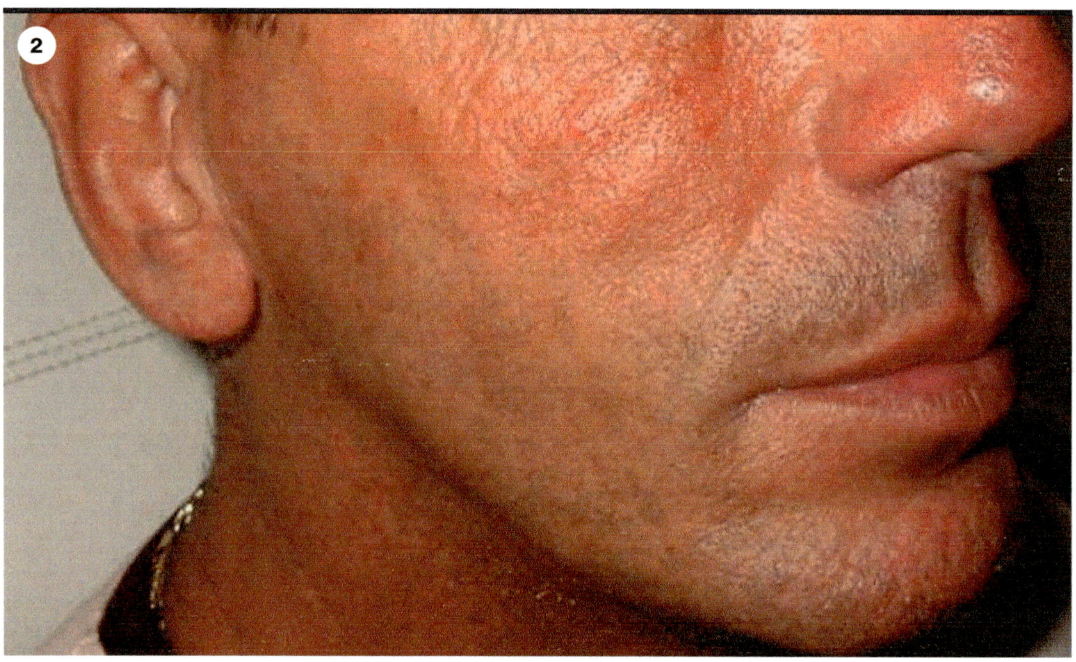

Figure 21.2
Same patient with normal lighting

Note that it is more challenging to visualize nodules using a direct flash light
Images courtesy Fred Tjan.

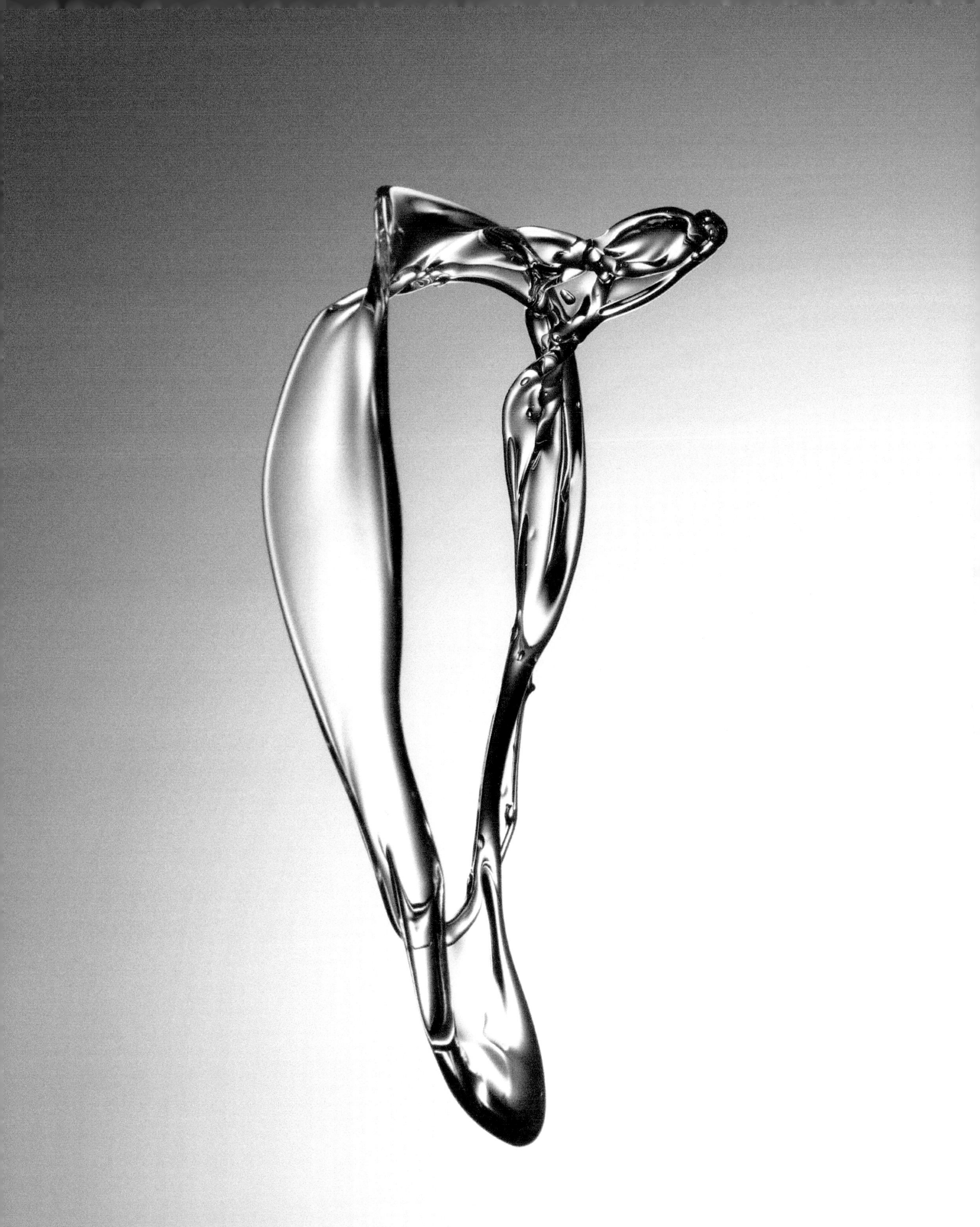

03

management of non-resorbable filler complications

Jonathan Kadouch, MD PhD
Pieter Siebenga, MD PhD
Tom Decates, MD PhD
Jani van Loghem, MD PhD

introduction

In this chapter we will cover a more in-depth description of granulomas, since granuloma formation is the most important problem that is seen with non-resorbable filler complications. Three different types of granulomas are described (cystic, edematous and sclerosing granulomas).

Different types of non-resorbable filler products are described; silicone oil, Polyacrylamide hydrogel (Aquamid), Polyalkylimide gel (Bio Alcamid), PMMA, HEMA, EMA, HME, PTFE, paraffin.
Complication management of especially silicone oil, Aquamid and Bio-Alcamid are described.

granulomas

3.1 Granulomas

Granulomas after STF injections are rare but can cause devastating and disfiguring effects to the affected patient. The clinical appearance is more pronounced with permanent STFs than with resorbable STFs and their persistence is longer if not treated adequately.[2] Currently, permanent STFs have been prohibited for use in many countries because of the risk of these severe late immunologic reactions.

As hyaluronic acid (HA) is a large human molecule (about 3-7 MDa)[145], it has a very low risk of inducing granuloma formation. However, cross-linking of HA molecules changes the 3D structure and therefor increases risk of foreign body reactions. The use of low molecular weight HA products may also increase risk of granuloma formation. Calcium hydroxylapatite (CaHA) is a human mineral and is not crosslinked for production of Radiesse. This product currently seems to have the lowest risk of granuloma formation among all STF products on the market.[2,146]

In case of granuloma formation after STF injection, phagocytosis is not successful because of remaining STF material in the tissue. After this chronic inflammation commences. In an attempt to isolate the STF when it cannot be eliminated otherwise, macrophages aggregate to form multinucleated giant cells and other immune cells enter into the area finally resulting in the formation of a granuloma.[2]

Phagocytosis has three phases:

01 Recognition of the foreign material and attachment to the cell membrane of the leukocyte (macrophage).

02 Engulfment and endocytosis. Pseudopods from the macrophage extend around the foreign material, ultimately forming an intracellular vacuole.

03 Degradation. By release of enzymes like collagenase and hyaluronidase and the release of superoxide ions and production of hydrogen peroxide, the foreign material is degraded and metabolized.

The generation of a granulomatous foreign body reaction (GFBR) is a 'normal', physiological response from the host to any foreign body. All STF agents used for soft-tissue augmentation are thought to elicit some degree of granulomatous inflammatory reaction following injection.[2,148] To a certain point this is considered to be part of a normal physiological response.[2,149]

A GFBR, or 'granuloma', is a histological diagnosis based on the pathologist's finding of:

- Histiocytes
- Multinucleated giant cells
- Lymphocytes
- Marked fibrosis
- Possibly the presence of a foreign body

GFBR can be classified according to a severity grading system and/or into different clinicohistological phenotypes. Duranti proposed a 4-point grading system for the severity of GFBR (Figure 24).[150] A genuine sarcoid-type (grade IV) GFBR, or 'granuloma', is predominantly composed of histiocytes/macrophages and giant cells encapsulating STF particles.[2,150] Lemperle and Lombardi proposed a classification of GFBR into different clinical and/or histological subtypes.[2, 151] Depending on the type of STF, different types of FBGs can arise.[2]

01

Cystic granulomas are caused by injected gels such as collagens and HA products. Clinical signs may include elevation, fluctuation (sterile abscess), redness, and induration. Cystic granulomas are usually small and superficial, they occur within the first year, and disappear spontaneously within another year. They are surrounded by a significant number of giant cells.

02

Edematous granulomas are caused by artificial fluids such as silicone and polyacrylamides. They appear suddenly years after injection with extensive swelling and are surrounded and infiltrated by mononuclear and inflammatory cells.

03

Sclerosing granulomas are caused by particulate injectables composed of PMMA, PLLA, PHMA, CaHA or dextran microspheres. They occur generally 6 months to 3 years after implantation and are visible, often bluish confined nodules. Histologically, the STF is infiltrated by many macrophages and giant cells, fibroblasts, and collagen fibers but few inflammatory cells.

granulomas

Figure 22
Classification of granulomatous foreign-body reactions by F. Duranti et al.

Images courtesy Jonathan Kadouch, MD PhD.

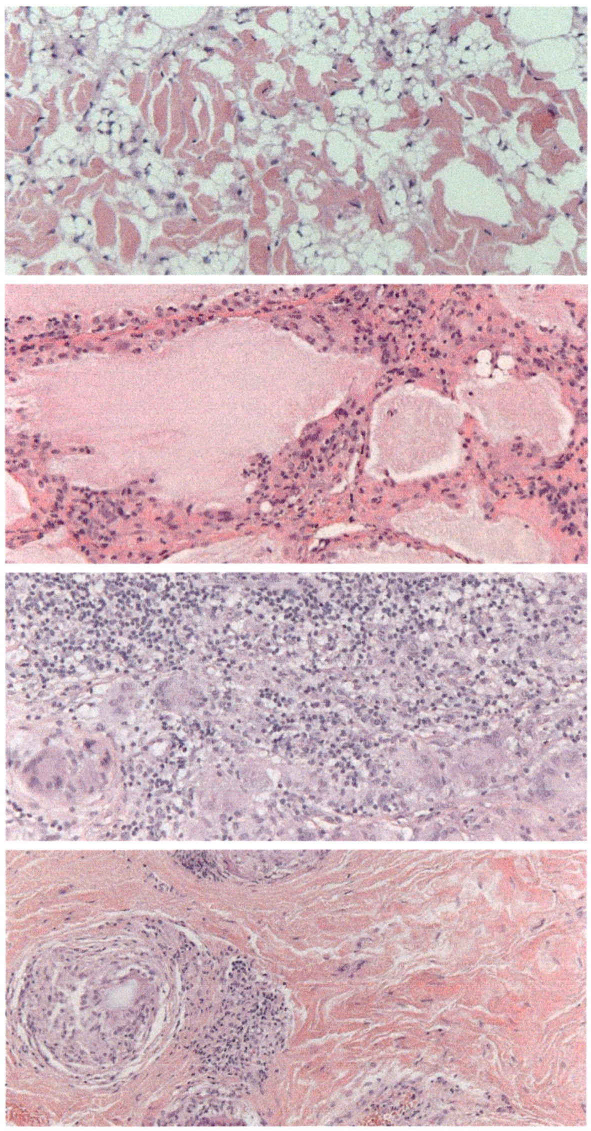

Grade I
Slight inflammatory reaction with few inflammatory cells, composed predominantly of histiocytes (macrophages), lymphocytes and plasma cells

Grade II
Clear inflammatory reaction with one or two multinucleated giant cells

Grade III
More multinucleated giant cells, the presence of lymphocytes and fibrous tissue with other inflammatory cells

Grade IV
A clear foreign-body reaction showing granulomas with encapsulated implants

Symptoms of a GFBR or granuloma include recurrent swelling, discoloration (redness), tenderness and sometimes even tissue destruction and open wounds. However, the extensiveness of the (histological) granulomatous reaction on STFs does not necessarily correlate with the clinical findings. Grade III of IV GFBRs can be found histologically, with clinically few or no symptoms, and vice versa.[187] Treatment of a GFBR is not necessary in healthy people without symptoms. Treatment should only be ensued following clear clinical symptoms such as redness and swelling in the face.

The exact pathophysiology of STF-induced GFBR, or 'STF granulomas', has yet to be elucidated.
Current insights differentiate several steps in host reaction on biomaterial implantation. Within minutes after implantation, host plasma components such as albumin, fibrinogen, fibronectin, lipids, sugars, ions and platelets are absorbed on the surface of the implant.[152-154] Platelets and other components of the coagulation cascade induce clot formation, which also functions as the provisional matrix around the biomaterial. Platelet adhesion and activation, and the release of pro-inflammatory cytokines, chemokines and growth factors induce sequentially the acute and chronic inflammatory responses on the implanted material. Damage-associated molecular patterns (DAMPs), pathogen-associated molecular patterns (PAMPs) and alarmins present at the implantation site activate macrophages, leukocytes and dendritic cells through pattern recognition receptors (PRRs), Toll-like receptors (TLRs) and C-type lectin.[54,152,155-158]
In the acute phase, the recruited neutrophils attempt to degrade the biomaterial through phagocytosis and the release of proteolytic enzymes, reactive oxygen species (ROS) and neutrophil extracellular traps (NETs, consisting of granular proteins, elastase, histones and chromatin DNA).[49,148,152] NETs are usually involved in trapping pathogens and prevention of infection spread.

The release of immune-regulatory signals by neutrophils attracts monocytes, macrophages, immature DCs and lymphocytes, promotes monocytes differentiation into pro-inflammatory "M1"-type macrophages secreting pro-inflammatory cytokines (Interleukin (IL-) 1β, IL-6, tumor necrosis factor alpha (TNF-α)) and downregulates the presence and activity of neutrophils themselves. The next step in the healing process is a shift towards "M2"-type macrophages secreting anti-inflammatory cytokines (i.e. IL-10) and recruiting fibroblasts for effective tissue regeneration. The shift towards an anti-inflammatory "M2"-type healing response can be altered by specific characteristics of the implanted material. For example, particles larger than 5 μm require the presence of aggregated macrophages, or giant cells, to be phagocytosed.[159-161] Particles larger than 15 to 20 μm are generally not subject to ingestion by macrophages by true phagocytosis, but may be enclosed by giant cells. Failure of effective phagocytosis leads to a chronic inflammation pathway and granuloma formation, consisting of macrophages and giant cells, as well as a contiguous infiltrate of lymphocytes secreting pro-inflammatory cytokines (i.e. tumor necrosis factor alpha (TNF-α), interferon gamma (IFN-γ) and interleukin 12 (IL-12)).[152,162] Similarly, excessive production of NETs by neutrophils can impair healing and lead to a chronic inflammation and encapsulation.[152,160,161]

granulomas

In case of an excessive GFBR, or granuloma formation after injected STF, the STF is recognized by the host as foreign material. Different factors influence the likelihood of recognition as a foreign material:

01 Characteristics of the patient's immune system;

02 Use of STFs with unfavorable structural properties (e.g. particulate STFs with irregular surface);

03 Presence of impurities within the STF (like bacterial peptides);

04 Contamination of the STF with bacteria or other foreign material.

Numerous studies have been performed on the different structural properties of soft-tissue fillers (STFs), such as chemical composition, electrical charge, surface irregularities or particle size and the presence of contaminants, which are of known influence on host immune responses[2,49] For example, particles larger 20 μm are not phagocytosed[159,160], while small particle sizes (<20μm) are faster phagocytosed and thus result in a greater local inflammatory reaction, which may result into local necrosis.[49] Positively charged particles attract and/or activate macrophages[163], irregularly shaped particles elicit a longer-lasting inflammatory reaction and smooth surfaces induce formation of a thicker fibrous capsule around the material.[49,159,164,165] Hydrophilic polymer gels constantly exchange water with the surrounding host tissue.[57] They are highly biocompatible and easily penetrable by nutrients and waste products[166], making them a suitable matrix for bacterial growth. Hydrophobic particles favor fibronectin absorption and therefore cellular adhesion, thus promoting a pro-inflammatory response.[49]

Hyaluronic acid (HA) is a non-sulfated glycosaminoglycan and has gained popularity as STF over the past decade. HA is a major component of the extracellular matrix of the skin and plays a prominent role in the metabolism of the dermis, regulating tissue injury, accelerating tissue repair and controlling disease outcomes.[152,167,168] HA STFs vary in molecular size and the amount of chemical crosslinking, which is believed to influence the host immune response.[169,170] Several studies have suggested that low molecular weight HA (LMW-HA) is pro-inflammatory and triggers the immune-system[168], whereas high molecular weight HA (HMW-HA) is believed to have intrinsic anti-inflammatory properties due to its radical oxygen species-scavenging properties.[152,168] However, as HA for STF production is generally of bacterial origin (with lower molecular weights) and crosslinked with 1,4-butanediol diglycidyl ether (BDDE), the risks of recognition as foreign increase. BDDE can cause conformational changes resulting in an altered 3-dimentional shape of the HA molecules and residual BDDE may be present in the final product (impurities).
Also, few practitioners realize that hydrolytic degradation of polymeric biomaterials (e.g. HAs, polycaprolactone, polylactic acid) can release CO2 with a consequent decrease in local pH, damaging cells and inducing local necrosis.[152]

Lastly, it must be noted that particulate STFs like calcium hydroxylapatite (CaHA) demonstrate a different safety profile than gel-based STFs like HA.[60,169] The predominant adverse event for CaHA are nodules, rarely edema and swelling or signs of inflammation. For HA the inflammatory AEs are more predominant. These different STF-related properties can influence host immune response, and these insights promote researchers to investigate biomaterial physicochemical modification to tune the host immune response favoring integration and healing.

3.2 Non-resorbable fillers

Since Neuber reported about facial rejuvenation with autologous fat transfer in 1893,[84] a wide variety of injectable STF have emerged on the market. STF can be divided in 2 categories, depending on the duration of the STF in the body: resorbable and non-resorbable. This chapter will focus on the recognition and management of the permanent (non-resorbable) STFs. An overview of the permanent STFs on the market with their AE profile/microscopic features can be found in Table 4.

Table 4
Non-degradable soft tissue fillers

Soft tissue filler	Product	Adverse event or microscopic features [2, 3, 11]
Polydimethyl siloxilane (silicone oil)	Dermagen Silicex Silikon 1000 Adatosil 5000	Clumping, migration, chronic inflammation, or granulomatous reaction with pseudoxanthomatous containing translucent particles of birefringent silicone. Late siliconomas.
Polyacrylamide hydrogel (PAAG)	Aquamid Evolution Outline	Swelling at the injection site, often combined with tingling sensation and redness. Ecchymosis and gel accumulation. Pain, purulent secretion or cysts occurred. Late adverse events include localized permanent indurations, abscess formation and migration of the gel due to muscular activity or gravity. Microscopic findings: foreign body and palisading granulomatous reaction surrounding a large pool of basophilic foamy material with mucinous appearance.
Polyalkylimide gel	Bio-alcamid	Early adverse events include bruising, pain, swelling and modest inflammatory reaction. Late adverse events have been reported, such as late-onset edema, capsule formation, abscess formation, infection, migration, inflammatory nodules and foreign body granulomas. Microscopic: irregular encapsulation, dystrophic calcification, acute inflammation in relation to pools of alcian-blue-positive basophilic mucinous material.
PMMA in collagen or carboxymethyl-cellulose.	Artecoll	Swelling after implantation, long lasting redness, persistent pain, transparency of the product, lumpiness and nodule formation. Allergic reaction has occurred. Chronic inflammatory reaction and granuloma formations 1–10 years past treatment. Immediate necrosis and blindness have been reported.
Polymethylmethacrylate (copolymer HEMA and EMA) in hyaluronic acid	Dermalive	Swelling, redness, discoloration, formation of nodules. Keratoacanthoma-like reaction. Inflammatory nodules and long-term reports of granuloma reactions.

Continued on next page

non-resorbable fillers

Soft tissue filler	Product	Adverse event or microscopic features [2, 3, 11]
Hydroxyethyl methacrylate/ ethyl methacrylate		Granulomatous reaction with many giant cells engulfing polygonal translucent structures.
Poly-tetrafluoroethylene (PTFE)/expanded PTFE.		Migration. Acute inflammation with granulation tissue suggesting infection.
Paraffin		Mild and transient local nodules and infection. Pseudo-lymphoma besides paraffinomas. Facial nodules, cellulites, facial ulcerations and migration. Microscopic: foreign-body granulomatous reaction containing abundant vacuoles of large size.

Silicone

Silicone has been injected for over 50 years. For a long time, silicone was the only material used for cosmetic indications. Only since the late 1990s, products based on other materials have been developed. Other non-biodegradable products that gained widespread use from that time were polyacrylamide hydrogel and polyalkylimide gel. Liquid injectable silicon oil for soft tissue augmentation was introduced in the late 1950s.[14,92-95] It then had a viscosity of 350 cS (100 cS is the viscosity of water), whereas the currently marketed silicone gels Silikon 1000® (Alcon Laboratories, Fort Worth, Texas) and Adatosil 5000® (Bausch & Lomb, Rochester, N.Y.) have a viscosity of 1000 cS with a certain amount of low molecular polymer to keep them pliable.[2] Histologically, silicone fluid forms only a very-thin-walled fibrous capsule, which means that migration, due to gravitational forces, along the fascia and muscle planes may occur.[53]

Polyacrylamide hydrogel

Polyacrylamide hydrogel (Aquamid®, Contura International A/S, Denmark) has been used extensively for soft tissue augmentation and body contouring for the past 20 years.[89] Aquamid is a biocompatible and nonabsorbable hydrogel consisting of 97.5% water and 2.5% cross-linked polyacrylamide.[90] After injection, Aquamid® undergoes cell infiltration and integration into tissues between weeks 1 and 8 where a fine fibrous capsule forms around the product.[53,91]

Polyalkylimide gel

Polyalkylimide gel (Bio-alcamid®, Polymekon, Milan, Italy) is a non-biodegradable hydrogel polymer which is an alkylic resin. It consists of 96% pyrogen-free water and 4% alkylimide-amide groups. It is considered to be a permanent STF due to the stability of its components and its resistance to hydrolysis.[86] Within 6 weeks after injection, the Bio-alcamid® becomes encapsulated with a thin collagen capsule.[87,88]

With respect to safety of permanent STFs a number of prospective, retrospective and case reports have been published.[85] Non-resorbable fillers may lead to unforeseen late-onset AEs that may be more difficult to resolve. For example, in 1991 the FDA prohibited the use of silicon oil due to the evidence of severe side effects such as allergies, inflammatory reactions, and granulomatous reactions. Alternatives with a nonpermanent profile are available and should first be considered in the case of volume loss or facial rejuvenation.

Prevention and management of adverse events after non-resorbable filler injection

Prevention

By Dutch law, it is prohibited to use non-resorbable filler for any purpose other than reconstructive. In our opinion, the only way to prevent non-resorbable filler-related AEs is to completely avoid these products, since they pose an increased, life-time risk of AEs. Besides, extra caution should be taken to inject a second filler in an area that has previously been injected (or suspected) with a non-resorbable filler. This may lead to the activation of immunological responses resulting in the onset of a granulomatous foreign body reaction (GFBR).

Management

Acute AEs after permanent STF injection will encompass the same treatment as explained in the previous chapters and will not be further elaborated on in this chapter. Subacute AEs is a somewhat vague description, but usually occurs after a couple of weeks and is mostly due to immunological reactions (infection or hypersensitivity). Abscess formation can be acute or subacute which must be incised and drained of its content. The content must then be sent for bacterial microscopy and culture. Depending on the sensitivity, antibiotic treatment should be started immediately. Abscesses may also occur as late-onset AEs and are then usually 'sterile' abscesses.

Late-onset, or delayed adverse events of non-degradable STFs include swelling, nodules, abscesses and/or ulcerations and GFBR at the site of the initial injection or at distant sites because of migration of the filler particles.[2,30,47,50,53,98-100] The onset of the AEs can start several months to several years after injection. Permanent products pose several challenges as they remain in the body which complicates the treatment of the AEs.

Delayed adverse events are more common with non-resorbable fillers. The host tissue can induce a foreign body response leading to the encapsulation of the non-resorbable filler, which may then lead to the formation of a granuloma. Clinically, GFBRs are often characterized by red, tender nodules, hyperpigmentation, scar formation, or suppurative abscesses.[2,53,98,101-105] Although the etiology of the granuloma formation remains unclear, various theories have been hypothesized, such as the implantation of a large quantity of fillers, impurities in the filler agent, irregularities in the surface of the filler, and the impact of biofilms.[106]

When a GFBR is suspected, the treating physician should always consider referring the patient to a centre which is specialized in the treatment of these types of complications.

When granulomatous adverse events do occur, they should be managed systemically (Figure 23). There have been reports of spontaneous disappearance of the granulomas, but one should not expect this.[14,97] Local or systemic drugs are the first choice of treatment. If the swelling is fluctuating, it should be considered as an abscess and be treated the way it has been described previously. If there is less or no fluctuation, systemic administration of antibiotics should be started. Oral administration of minocycline 100mg BID have led to successful remission of silicon induced granulomas.[96] Macrolides have effectively been found to treat inflammatory reactions, prevent the formation of a biofilm, and suppress foreign body responses by up-regulating the production of anti-inflammatory mediators.[107-110] Systemic or intralesional corticosteroid (triamcinolone - Kenalog 20–40mg/ml intralesional) as adjuvant therapy can be considered. The corticosteroid should be injected into the cellular tissue surrounding the implant and aids in the control of the inflammatory processes surrounding the filler.[73] However, both drug therapies do not remove the filler. Intralesional laser therapy (ILT) is able to remove STFs in a minimally invasive way.[36,56,111] Patients are treated with a diode laser, developed and used for endovenous laser treatments, which is introduced in the filler pocket. During the treatment a softening of the product is expected. Directly after the softening of the filler, the heat-liquefied filler can be (partly) squeezed out by manual compression, through an 18-gauge needle entry point or through a small incision made by a no. 11 scalpel.[56] Delicate areas can be pre-treated with corticosteroid injections to avoid skin burns.

non-resorbable fillers

If the product is not clinically easily felt or seen, the fiber insertion can be performed under ultrasound guidance. Intradermal anesthesia at the skin entry point is commonly used.[56] Surgical excision should be used as a last resort. Especially in the case of silicone this should be avoided, since complete excision is difficult due to the silicone's tentacle-like shoots into the tissue. Finally, a total flap can be considered.

Figure 23
Algorithm for management of granulomatous AEs

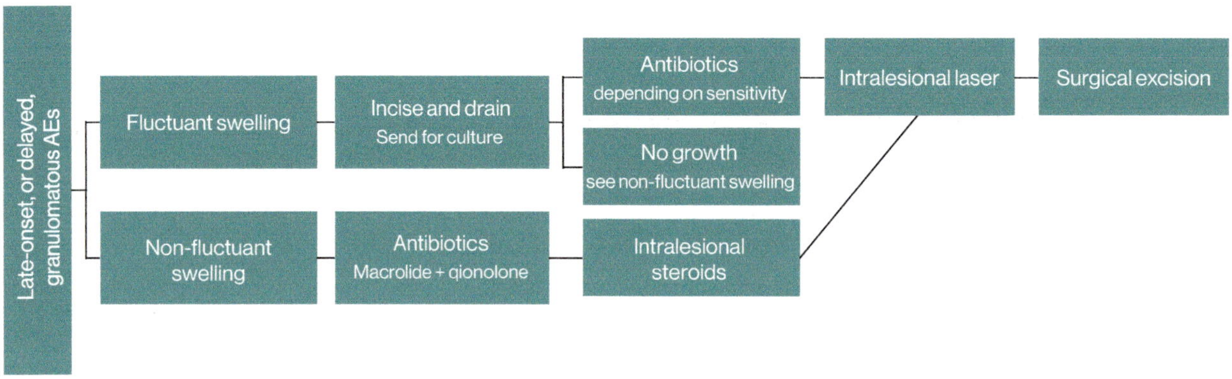

Non-resorbable fillers pose a permanent risk to complications. Knowledge on how to manage non-resorbable filler complications is essential to improve patient safety.

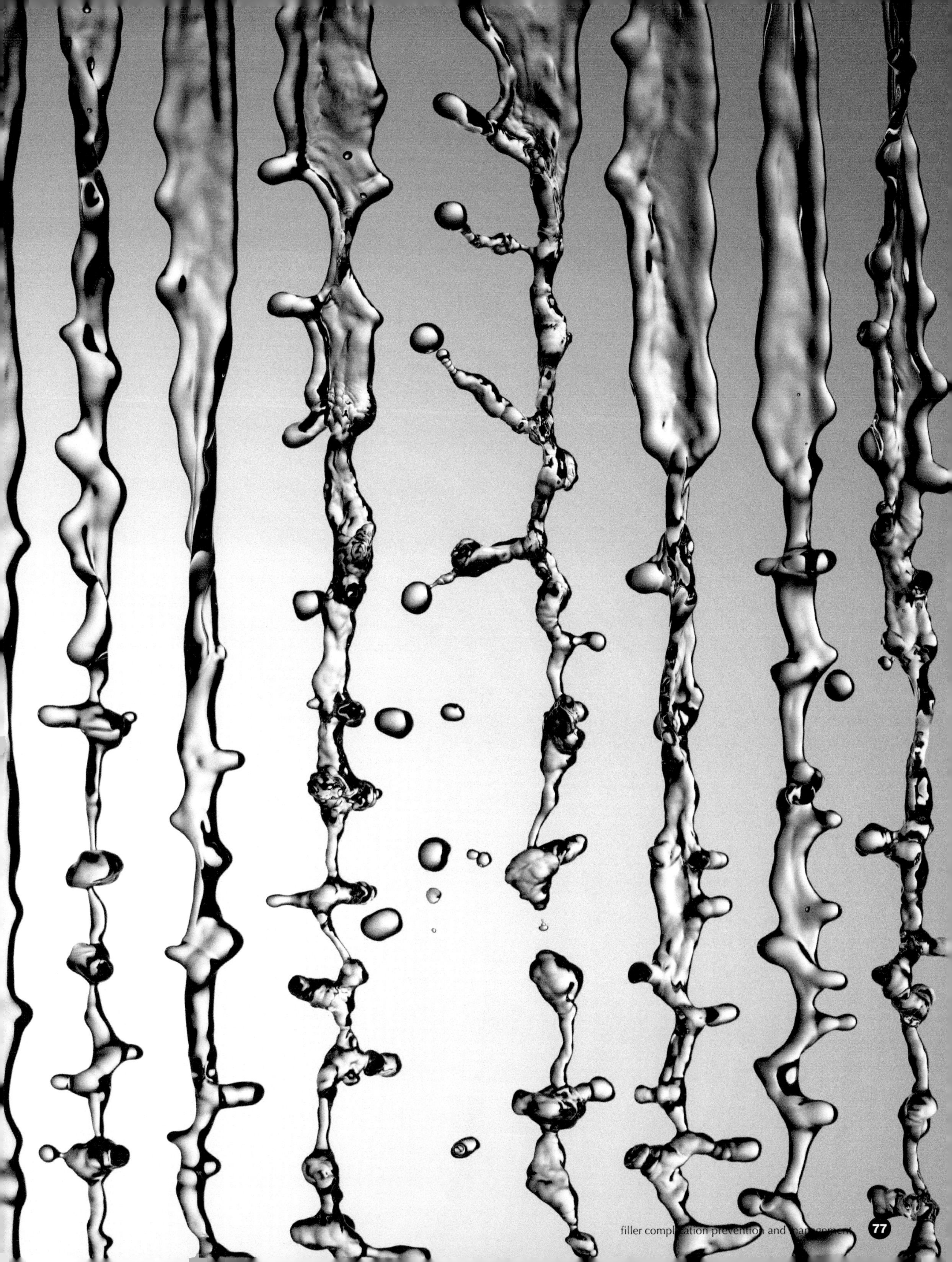

04
ultrasound imaging in filler complications

Peter Velthuis, MD PhD
Leonie Schelke, MD PhD
Tom Decates, MD PhD

introduction

Ultrasound devices have become accessible and necessary devices in aesthetic clinics. In this chapter, the multidisciplinary group of specialized physicians working in the Filler Complications Unit at the Erasmus Medical Center outpatient department of dermatology is sharing important insights in prevention and management of soft tissue filler complications.

Prevention: scanning for anatomic variations of vasculature, diagnosing possible non-resorbable fillers.

Management: injection of hyaluronidase under direct ultrasound guidance

ultrasound imaging in filler complications

4.1 Ultrasound imaging in filler complications

Sonography or ultrasound imaging is rapidly becoming popular in many areas of medicine. In particular the notion that the new, small and portable devices can be applied in so called point-of-care testing has boosted the use of ultrasound imaging. It has become an indispensable tool in emergency units because it can rapidly detect critical conditions such as ectopic pregnancy, leaking abdominal aorta, etc. Ultrasound can also help in diminishing procedural complications for instance by the placement of central venous lines and thorax drains. Because of all these benefits the hand-held sonographic devices have been nick-named the stethoscope of the future.

In dealing with filler complications ultrasound imaging is a powerful tool. In this area of medicine, it can have several functions (Table 5).

Table 5
Ultrasound imaging in filler complications

01	Preventive tissue scanning for variations in vascular anatomy
02	Preventive tissue scanning for prior injected filler substances
03	Detection of filler type involved in the complication
04	Detection of type of adverse reaction (inflammatory panniculitis, abscess, granuloma)
05	Ultrasound guided treatment in hyaluronidase injections or intralesional laser treatment (ILT)

Filler images under ultrasound

Soft tissue fillers can be divided into hydrophilic (water containing) and hydrophobic (no water containing). The former is black (= an-echoic) or grayish (= hypo-echoic) on the monitor. The latter is bright gray or white (= hyper-echoic). Some fillers have mixed echogenicity. Table 6 lists them all. Finally, one has to realize that structures can have the same echogenicity as the surrounding tissue (iso-echoic). In that case the filler can only be detected by moving the probe in order to get a dynamic image and by subsequently recognizing the difference in texture.

Hyaluronic Acid (HA) fillers are gels. These contain water, rendering them an-echoic. The ones with high G-prime are easily seen after injection as an-echoic oval shaped pockets (Figure 27). Low G-prime HA filler are less easily seen, because these mingle with the tissue. The non-resorbable hydrophobic fillers such as poly methyl methacrylic acid (PMMA) and liquid silicone give rise to reflection of almost all ultrasound waves. This leads to a band-like hyper-echoic picture. In case of liquid silicone this image is homogeneous very-small granular, which is also known as 'snowstorm' appearance. In PMMA the fine-granular hyperechoic band is heterogenous, being mingled with course granular structures. In both cases the reflection of the ultrasound waves is so intense that no waves pass the layer of the subcutaneous that is filled with the filler substance. This reflection blocks any imaging below the filler, giving rise to the artifact known as 'posterior shadowing' (Figure 25). This artefact is helpful in spotting the filler location.

The bio-stimulatory hydrophobic fillers (CaHA, poly-caprolactone) are hydrophobic substances suspended in gels in order to permit injection. Direct after injection these fillers appear as hypo-echoic grayish areas interspersed with hyper-echoic particles. In due time the gel is resorbed and with this the ultrasound image of these fillers will change. Eventually when new collagen is being produced, a subcutaneous iso-echoic area is formed. The area filled can only be detected because it is much more homogeneous than its environment. It is the difference in texture that makes identification possible.

Over time the images of all fillers, also the HA ones, tend to change in echogenicity, becoming more and more grayish and sometimes eventually iso-echoic.

Table 6

List of hydrophilic and hydrophobic soft tissue fillers

01	Hydrophilic	Hyaluronic acid	(various brands)
		Polyacrylamine	(Aquamid®)
		Polyalkylimide	(Bio-Alcamid®)
02	Hydrophobic	Polyacrylmethacrylate	(Artecoll®, Dermalive®)
		Liquid silicone	(Various brands)
03	Mixed	Calcium hydroxylapatite	(Radiesse®)
		Poly-caprolactone	(Ellanse®)
		Poly-L-lactic acid	(Sculptra)

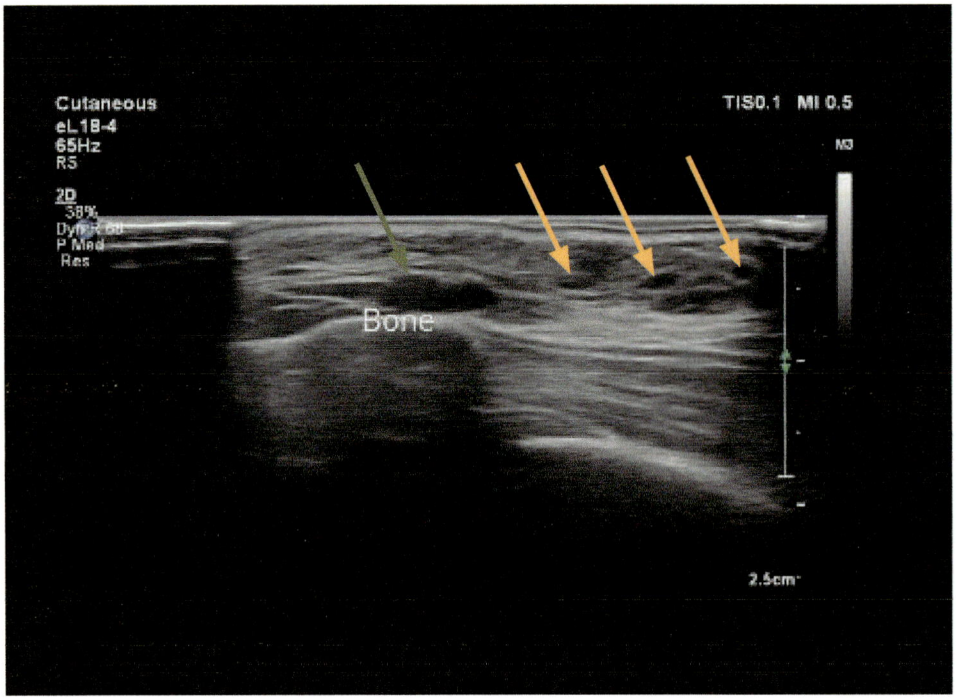

Figure 24
Hyaluronic acid filler

Three an-echoic pockets (yellow arrows) placed in the subcutis of the midface area and one bigger deposit at the periostium (green arrow).
Image courtesy Tom Decates, MD PhD

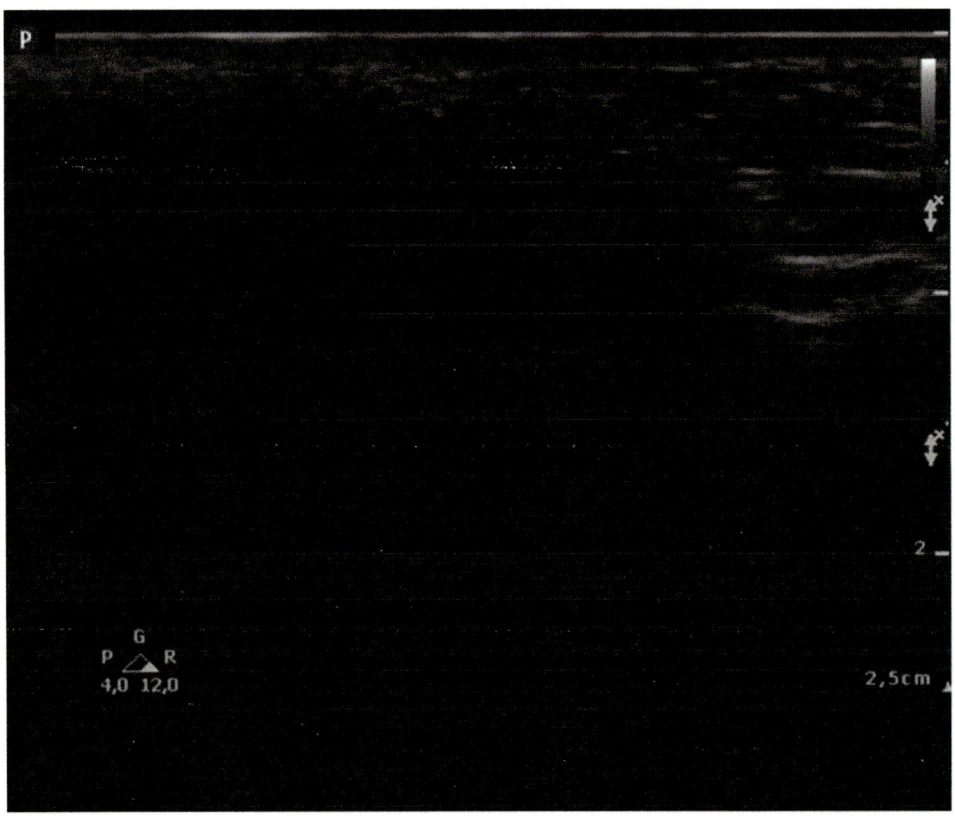

Figure 25
PMMA filler

A major part of this figure (middle and left side) shows a small heterogeneous hyper-echoic band with posterior shadowing. The band consists of small granules and somewhat larger coarse granular structures. On the right side a small area of normal subcutaneous skin is visible.
Image courtesy Tom Decates, MD PhD

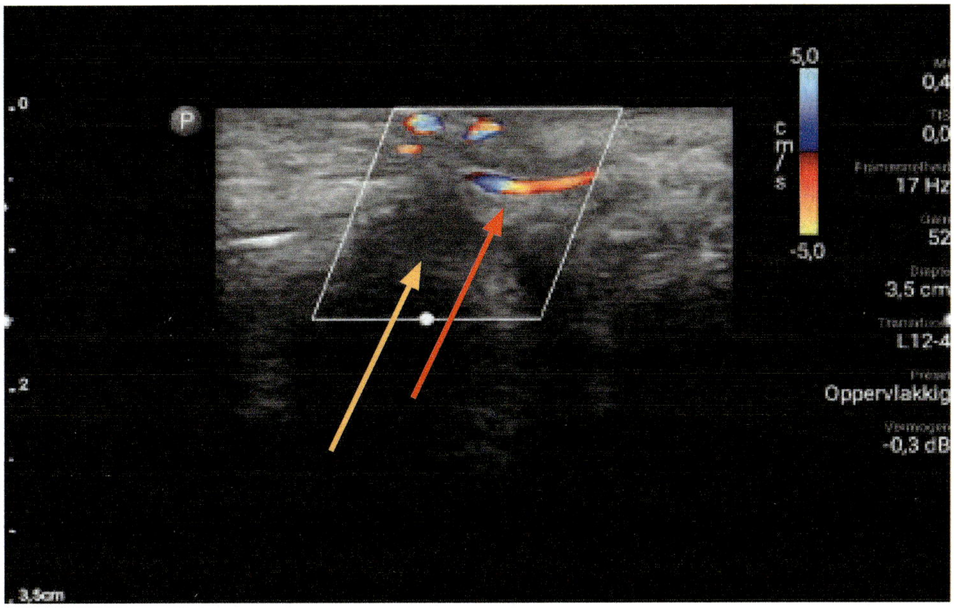

Figure 26
Doppler image of vascular adverse event

Note the distended artery with both blue and red colors, indicating both blood flow away as wel towards the transducer (red arrow). A deposit of hypoechoic material is seen to the left of the artery (yellow arrow). Image courtesy Tom Decates, MD PhD

Prevention of complications: pre-treatment assessment

Many clients do not recall filler being previously injected or are inclined to deny having had any. Knowing all of the above makes a pre-treatment assessment of the face with the object to spot previous fillers, possible. This will lead to an honest conversation with the client and assessment of the risk when injecting new fillers.

Another objective of pre-treatment ultrasonic assessment of the face is to identify variations in the position of anatomical structures. This will help to avoid injections into arteries or other delicate structures. We* have observed compression of the infra-orbital nerve with an HA filler giving rise to severe pain, which resolved instantly after hyaluronidase injection. Also, we have seen that it is relatively easy to inadvertently deliver filler material inside a superficial lying parotid gland while injecting near the mandibular angle.

Most cases of arterial blockage after filler injections concern the facial artery and its subsequent branches near the mouth. Other areas may be involved. We have seen pre-necrotic skin on the forehead after temporal injections with occlusion of the frontal branch of the superficial temporal artery, on the lateral cheek after occlusion of the transverse facial artery and in the oral cavity after injections inside the submental artery in a patient being injected on the inferior mandibular ramus. The vascular adverse event (VAE) feared most is the one causing vision loss. These injections mainly concern the angular artery, the arteries on the nose and the supraorbital and supratrochlear arteries. All arteries in the face are prone to variant courses, most notably when surgery has been performed priorly.
A thorough assessment of the area to be treated before the treatment itself will help to prevent problems like this.

*We is the group of doctors at the 'complication filler' office hours at Erasmus Medical Center Department of Dermatology. These doctors are: Tom Decates, Armanda Onderdijk, Leonie Schelke, Peter Velthuis, Jonathan Kadouch, Hajo Bruining and Lizenka Adriaanse

ultrasound imaging in filler complications

Ultrasound guided injections to resolve complications in hyaluronic acid fillers

Many of the complications with HA fillers that we see on our filler consultation hours at Erasmus MC (Rotterdam, The Netherlands) are created by flaws in technique. These concern nodules where either too much substance was injected, or the injection was too superficial. Also, intramuscular injection has led to migration of a product. Also, filler with high G-prime under thin skinned areas such as the lower eyelids or areas with little or no subcutaneous space such as the forehead are referred frequently. In most cases the physician had already injected hyaluronidase once or several times. After identifying the causative filler accumulation, we again perform an injection with hyaluronidase, but now under ultrasound guidance. We are successful in almost every case with 15-75 units. Apparently delivering the enzyme exactly in the HA filler substance has a much better effect that injecting here and there in the blind.

For ultrasound guided injections there must be a straight line from physician to the ultrasound monitor with in the middle the patient's problem area covered by the ultrasound probe. The needle to deliver the hyaluronidase needs to be thick enough to be detected by the ultrasound device. A needle of 25G or lower is recommended. This way, the doctor can see both the patient and the monitor at the same time. With experience, the doctor does not need to observe his hand but follows what happens on the monitor and adjusts the position of the probe when necessary.

This method is especially successful in cases of arterial occlusion. In those cases, the ultrasound monitor shows dilated collateral arteries, an image which we tentatively called 'the Medusa head'. In the middle of this Medusa head the anechoic HA filler can be identified. Injecting that spot with a small amount of hyaluronidase (50-100 units), sometimes repeated 1-2 times after 15 and 30 minutes, almost invariably leads to immediate restoration of the blood flow. In many instances we have seen that more than one artery is blocked. Apparently smaller parts of the HA filler mass may come loose and can travel to a more distant spot. So, it is important to follow the complete course of the blood flow in all the subsequent branches of the blocked arteries.

Other filler complications

In case of an inflammatory adverse event ultrasound imaging can make some distinctions. Panniculitis is depicted by hyper-echogenicity of the subcutaneous fat. Abscess formation is clearly visible as a hyperechoic mass surrounded by anechoic fluid. Edema, fibrosis, granulomas , infected threads, resorbable sutures and other objects can be distinguished by sonography. Most granulomas appear as hypoechoic, ill-delimited structures with heterogenous content and slight acoustic shadowing. However, we have found that it is sometimes difficult to differentiate between a hydrophilic filler itself and foreign body granuloma formation as a reaction to a filler. In the case of polyalkylamide for instance, we are frequently surprised that hypoechoic material, presumably containing a lot of water, cannot easily be taken out after stab incision and skin compression. These and other issues such as the way fillers integrate in the tissue over time and the way in which fillers migrate in the tissue after injection are open for investigation.

The ultrasound device

Portable ultrasound machines with 10-12 MHz probes are available for less than 10.000 euro/dollars. These offer good quality imaging of the first 4-6 cm under the skin surface. The color doppler (duplex mode) enables to detect bi-directional blood flow. Most of these machines have presets to facilitate their use. One does not have to be an expert radiologists to engage in ultrasound imaging of the face. It is however not so easy to find your way in interpreting the pictures built of various grey scales that fill the monitor. Moreover, sonography as an imaging tool is much different from other imaging techniques in the sense that it is not static but dynamic. The physician moves the probe over the area to be investigated by sliding from one side to the other, rotating around a subcutaneous object or tilting slightly to depict an object from various angles. All the time with the objection to create a 3-dimesional mental picture of the structures below the skin.

Despite all these hurdles we have found that with an intense two day hands-on training one can understand the basic of ultrasound and use this imaging technique to avoid and treat filler complications.

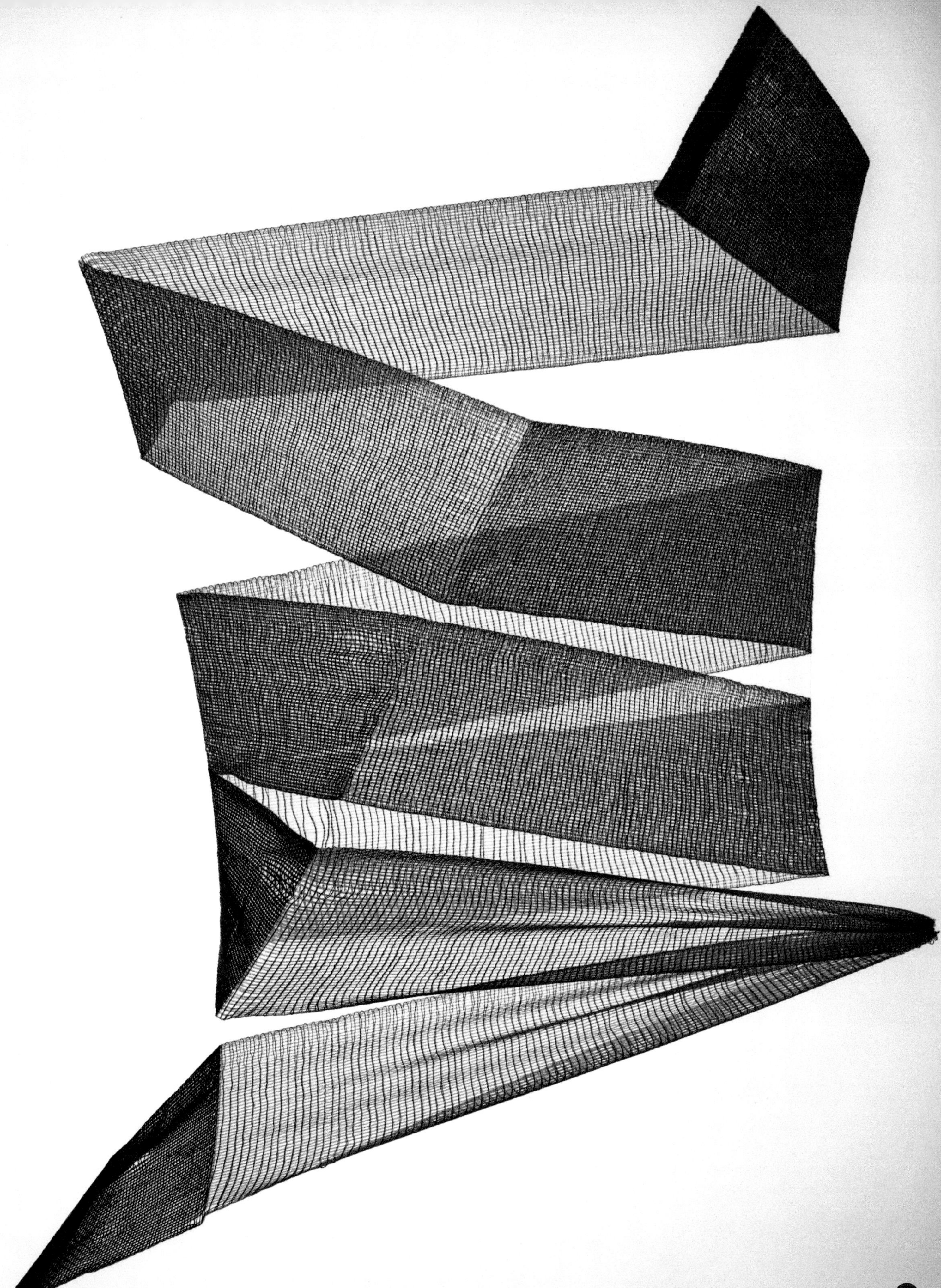

05
appendix

Pieter Siebenga, MD PhD
Benoit Hendrickx, MD PhD
Tom Decates, MD PhD
Jani van Loghem, MD PhD

introduction

In this appendix we add some valuable information for the aesthetic practitioner. Firstly, we share what we have in our complications management box; the UMA filler first aid kit. Then, we discuss hyaluronidase and give some extra background information.

We discuss post treatment scarring, different scar types (atrophic scars, hypertrophic scars, keloid scars, widespread (stretched) scars, scar contractures and acne scars). We discuss laser therapy in general terms and how lasers can assist in STF complication management.

uma filler first aid kit

5.1 UMA filler first aid kit

Nothing scares a physician more than an unexpected serious adverse event. The attending physician is expected to exude confidence while the situation is getting more demanding with every minute passing. It is difficult to remember the treatment algorithms and to calculate drug doses. While theoretical and practical training of acute settings is deemed essential, it is generally undertaken on voluntary basis. The authors believe all aesthetic physicians should refresh their knowledge of emergency treatment techniques and prepare themselves with therapeutic guidelines. Along the line of these preparations, we also believe that each clinic should equip itself with a filler first aid kit for acute situations.

Patients requiring immediate therapy will need appropriate monitoring and adequate application of systemically acting drugs. Diagnostic equipment as well as equipment for monitoring the respiratory and cardiovascular systems should be available. Clear therapeutic algorithms are the endpoint of proper emergency management (e.g., restoration of vital functions or reversing blindness).

Acute blindness, peripheral vascular compromise and anaphylactic shock are complications that need direct medical attention. The UMA filler first aid kit is therefore mainly equipped with tools for the acute management these complications. An overview of the UMA Institute filler first aid kit is depicted in Table 7. Handheld flow charts should be included and updated with the latest insights. At UMA Clinic, we have included a flowchart for edema/allergic reaction/anaphylactic shock, angio-edema after IV therapy, acute infection/abscess, vascular occlusion (HA and CaHA), and acute blindness (HA and CaHA).

Table 7
Overview of UMA Institute filler first aid kit

Item	Amount	Drug	Amount
Blood pressure meter	1	Saline 10ml vials	5
Stethoscope	1	Lidocaine 2% 10ml vials	5
Tourniquet	1	Hyaluronidase 1500U	4
3ml luer lock syringes	5	Anesthetic eye drops	1
10ml luer lock syringes	1	Timolol 0.5% eyedrops	1
18G needles	5	Adrenalin Epipen	1
27G, 38mm injection needles	5	Adrenaline 1ml vial	2
30G, 13mm needles	5	Tavegyl 1mg/ml 2ml vial	1
18G intravenous cannulas	2	Tavegyl 1mg tablets	10
IV needle stickers	2	Fraxiparine 9.500 IE anti-Xa/ml vial	1
IV tubing	1	Aspirin 500mg tablets	10
25G, 38mm TSK steriglide cannulas	5	Tadalafil 20mg tables	2
Gauzes 10x10cm, sterile, 5 pieces	5	Prednisolone 30 mg tablets	10
Alcohol swabs	5	Dexamethasone 4mg/ml 1ml vial	3
Medical tape	1	Furosemide 10mg/ml 2ml vial	1
Wound swab for culture	1	Levocetrizine 5mg tablets	10

hyaluronidase

The UMA filler first aid kit lists the essential medical tools to have close at hand in case of filler complications. Scars, lasers, hyaluronidase, novel innovations, (Doppler) Ultrasound and their roles in complication management are discussed here.

5.2 Hyaluronidase

Hyaluronidase is an enzyme that can, temporarily and reversibly, depolymerise the polysaccharides of HA. Via hydrolyzing of the polysaccharides, at hexosaminidic β-1 through β-4 linkages, it leads to a degradation of the HA.[112] Hyaluronidase has an immediate effect, with only a half-life of two minutes. However, the duration until the effect becomes visible takes much longer, approximately 24 to 48 hours.[113-115]

Hyaluronidase needs to be stored at cool temperature (between 2–8°C, 35–46°F) to guarantee the stability of the product. Reconstitution is done with water of saline; the latter is most often chosen since it is more patient friendly upon injection. Depending on the indication hyaluronidase is reconstituted with 1 ml to 10 ml. High concentration of hyaluronidase is required when vascular occlusion is suspected or when a large volume of HA needs to be dissolved. Lower concentration may be used when small volume of HA needs to be dissolved with more precision. Once a vial of hyaluronidase is opened, it should be used immediately. Any unused content should be discarded afterwards. More information of the clinical particulars, pharmacological properties and pharmaceutical particulars can be found in the summary of product characteristics (SmPC). In STF vascular complications, off label use of lidocaine for reconstitution is often advocated due to its vasodilatory properties. Reconstitution in lidocaine 2% is advised in our algorithms as well.

Hyaluronidase can be derived from mammals (bovine or ovine, obtained from the tested), hookworms or leeches, or microbes.[117] Also, recombinant human hyaluronidase is on the market (Hylenex®, Halozyme Therapeutics, San Diego, USA) (King). Indications include the management of lumps, nodules, overcorrections and asymmetries after HA injection. Also, injection of a high concentration of hyaluronidase is required when vascular compromise is suspected, either due to intravascular injection or external compression.

Type I (IgE-mediated) or Type IV (T-cell mediated) allergic reactions have been described after injection with hyaluronidase. Bovine derived hyaluronidase has a higher incidence of allergic reactions due to its exogenous origin. A test patch is advised when hypersensibility is suspected with a dose of at least 8 units intradermally in the forearm and an observation period of at least 30 minutes. Patients with a wasp or bee allergy should always be tested first, since the venom of wasps and bees contains hyaluronidase which is the cause of the hypersensibility in some cases.[73]

Drugs, such as NSAIDs, anti-histamines and vitamin C are antagonists of hyaluronidase. Higher dosages are sometimes required in these cases to resolve the HA.

post-treatment scarring

5.3 Post-treatment scarring

Scar formation is rare after soft tissue filler treatment, but when it occurs, it can have a major impact on the quality of life. Fortunately, scars are often considered trivial, but they can be aesthetically unpleasant or even disfiguring. Accompanying symptoms may include itching, tenderness, pain, sleep disturbance, anxiety, depression, and disruption of daily activities.[120]

Scars can occur after an injury to the skin as a result of an operation, an accident or a skin disease. After the injury, wound healing occurs. A wound heals in three stages.

01 The inflammatory phase lasts one to four days from the onset of the wound. During this phase, the body cleans the wound, and the actual wound healing begins, producing scar tissue and collagen fibers.

02 The regeneration phase lasts from the fourth to the twenty-first day. Blood vessels, collagen fibers, lymph vessels and nerves will recover in this phase.

03 The maturation phase begins on the twenty-first day and can last a year (or more). In this phase there is a balance between the production and breakdown of collagen fibers. The scar becomes less red, more superficial and smoother.

Usually, an injury to the skin heals well. There will also be a 'normal' scar in the form of a thin, white line. When wound healing is disturbed, problems can arise, and the scar cannot heal properly. A disturbance in wound healing can have various causes, such as an infection, a poor general condition of the skin or poor circulation in the wound area. We distinguish a number of different scars:

01

Atrophic scars

In atrophic scars, the skin underneath the scar is reduced. The scar is often very thin and retracted.

02

Hypertrophic scars

Hypertrophic scars are wide, pink or dark pigmented scars. In a hypertrophic scar, too much collagen tissue has formed. Hypertrophic scars are raised above the skin, but stay within the boundaries of the original lesion.

03

Keloid scars

Keloid scars are similar to hypertrophic scars, but the proliferation of the scar tissue spreads beyond the boundaries of the original wound. Keloid scars usually develop after trauma and are more common in black people.

04

Widespread (stretched) scars

These type of scars usually appear post-surgery and gradually become stretched and widened. These scars are typically flat, pale, soft and symptomless scars often seen after surgery near joints. Striae are a variant of widespread scars in which there has been injury to the dermis and subcutaneous tissue, but the epidermis is intact. There is no elevation, thickening, or nodularity in mature wide- spread scars.[119]

05

Scar contractures

Scars that cross joints or skin creases at right angles are prone to develop shortening or contracture. Scar contractures occur when the scar is not fully matured, often tend to be hypertrophic, and are typically disabling and dysfunctional. They are common after burn injury across joints or skin concavities.

06

Acne scars

When acne heals, it can be accompanied by scars. The scars may be atrophic (a dimple in the skin) or the scars may be pigmented.

post-treatment scarring

Deciding whether to treat a scar or leave it alone depends on accurate diagnosis of scar type and scar site, accompanying symptoms, severity and stigma (how much is the patient disturbed?). It is best to leave most scars undisturbed for at least a year to mature. If treatment is preferred, one can chose for non-invasive or invasive treatment options. Non-invasive include compression therapy (such as pressure garments with or without gel sheeting); static and dynamic splints; acrylic casts; masks and clips; application of a variety of oils, lotions, and creams; antihistamine drugs; hydrotherapy; and psychosocial counselling and advice.[120,121] Silicon sheeting, with or without adhesive, has become popular. Massage therapy is often advocated but lacks evidence.

Invasive treatments include surgical excision and re-suture. Generally, revision should be considered only if the surgeon thinks that more favorable conditions for wound healing can be provided than on the first occasion (less inflammation, better technique). Intra-lesional corticosteroid injection[120] is widely used but is prone to complications (fat atrophy, dermal thinning, and pigment changes). Other treatments that have been advocated with variable outcomes include injections of fluorouracil, interferon gamma, and bleomycin, radiotherapy, laser therapy, and cryo-surgery.[122-127]

When such management plans are applied to specific scar types, certain patterns emerge:

01

Atrophic scars have been improved with chemical peels, cutaneous laser resurfacing, dermabrasion, punch excisions, and the use of soft tissue biological and alloplastic biological fillers.[119,128]

02

Treatment of **widespread scars** is mostly by revision surgery to narrow the width of the scar. Revised scars in anatomical sites subject to excessive tissue mobility such as limbs can benefit from splinting.[119,129]

03

Keloids It is important to distinguish between hypertrophic and keloid scars as inappropriate management can lead to recurrence and larger scars. Simple surgical excision of keloid scars has a 50%-80% risk of recurrence. A combination of surgery with either intralesional corticosteroid injection or radiotherapy has been the mainstay of treatment.[130,131] Other treatment options, either as mono- or combination treatment, include cryotherapy, compression therapy, silicone sheets, or 5-Fluorouracil 50 mg/ml (50-150 mg per dose, maximally 16 doses).

04

Hypertrophic scars may be treated with surgical excision. Chance of recurrence are present, but the incidence is lower than keloids.

05

For **scar contractures**, surgical release with splinting, acrylic casting, and compression therapy may be required. Full thickness and split or partial thickness skin grafts and, perhaps more effectively, local and free flaps are used for reconstruction of difficult and extensive care and contractures.[132]

06

Acne scars Multiple modalities for acne scarring treatment exist including microneedling (with or without PRP), lasers (nonfractional CO2 and erbium-doped:YAG (Er:YAG) lasers, as well as ablative fractional lasers,[133,134] chemical peels, and STF.

5.4 Basic principles for the use of laser therapy in complication management

Lasers (Light Amplification by the Stimulated Emission of Radiation) are devices that emit a single, coherent wavelength of electromagnetic radiation that is used to cut, coagulate, or ablate tissue.[135] Lasers are used in a variety of clinical applications commonly related to external structures that are easily reached, such as the skin and cornea, but may also be used for deeper structured (e.g., bronchial structures, gastrointestinal mucosa, and urinary tract). Light is electromagnetic radiation within the range of wavelength that is visible to the human eye. Medical lasers produce photons of electromagnetic energy that can be within, above, or below this range.

Different laser systems produce a variety of wavelengths of varying pulse duration and energy levels, each developed for a specific purpose. A thorough understanding of interactions between light and biologic tissue is critical for the selection of a laser device as well as the effective and safe use of it. With optimal laser settings, a laser can be aimed precisely to a target chromophore, while avoiding damage to healthy tissue. The authors strongly advice to read the user manual before you use the equipment.

When laser energy encounters tissue surface, energy can be absorbed, reflected, transmitted, or scattered. Absorption of light is necessary to exercise its effects on tissue (both beneficial and adverse). Molecules that absorb light are called chromophores. Frequently targeted chromophores in the skin are melanin, oxyhemoglobin, and water. Tattoo ink is another chromophore which is targeted often in laser therapy (Table 8). Clinically, light is absorbed into the target chromophore and converted to thermal energy, leading to heating and ultimately in the destruction of the chromophore [1]. Absorption of laser and light by various tissues are depicted in Figure 26. The optimal pulse duration is determined from the thermal relaxation time of the target chromophore. The thermal relaxation time is the time needed for the tissue temperature to return to its baseline temperature after heating.[135] If a tissue is heated for a period less than or equal to its thermal relaxation time, the accumulated heat and subsequent damage is confined to the target object, whereas if a target is heated for longer than its thermal relaxation time, heat conduction leads to heating of surrounding structures, possibly damaging the healthy tissue.

Table 8
Common chromophore targets in the skin

Chromophore	Light absorption range
Water	Infrared
Fat (adipocytes)	Near infrared
Sebaceous gland	Near infrared
Deoxyhemoglobin	Near infrared
Melanin	Ultraviolet > visible light >> near infrared
Aminolevulinic acid	Red, blue
Oxyhemoglobin	Bleu-green > yellow >> near infrared
Proteins	Ultraviolet
DNA, RNA	Ultraviolet

laser therapy

Figure 27
Absorption of laser and light by various tissues

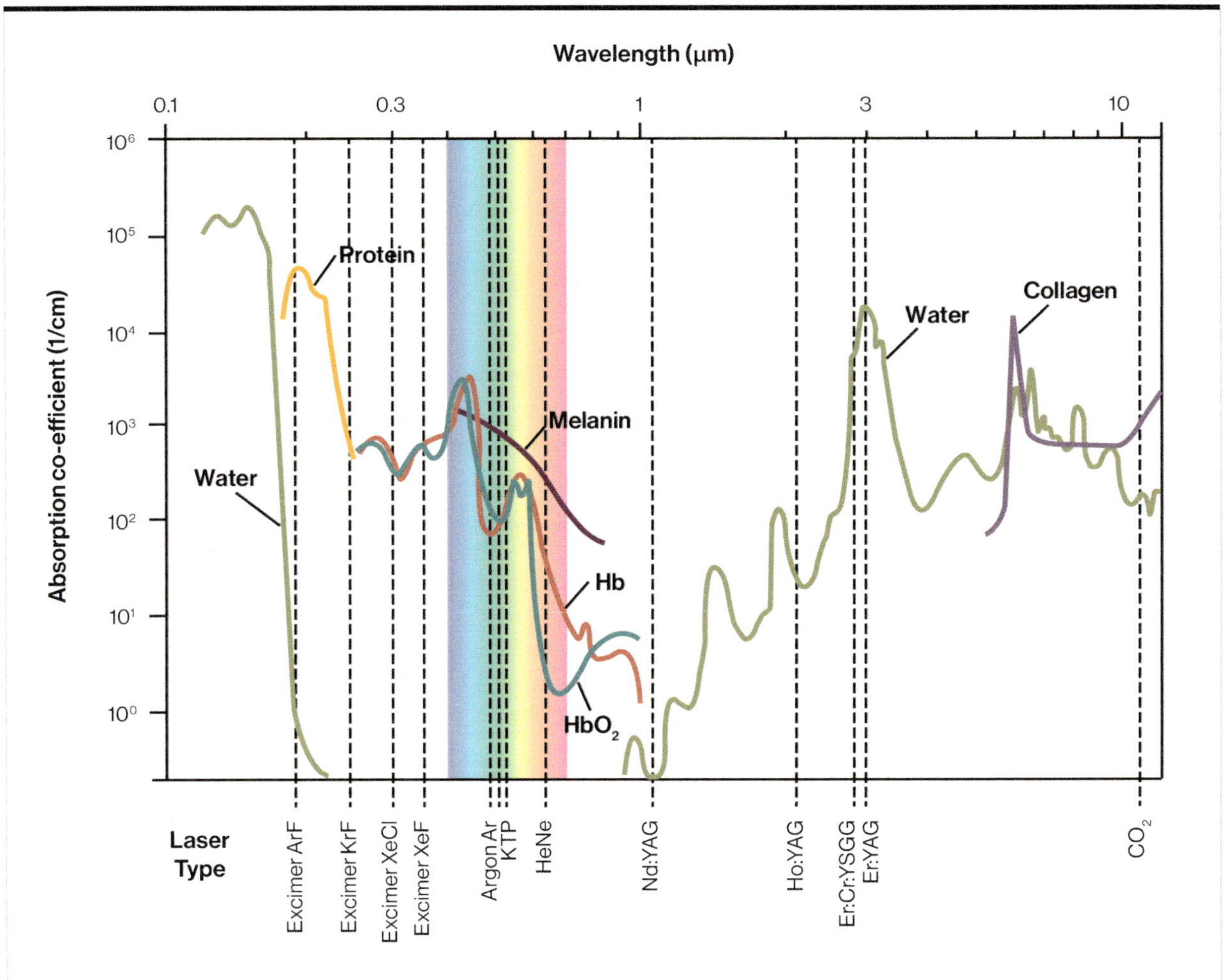

The effect of the interaction between the laser and tissue depends upon the active medium, wavelength, power density, properties of the target tissue, and duration of tissue exposure.[136] The wavelength of the laser beam determines the degree of tissue penetration, absorbed energy, and scattered energy. The longer the wavelengths, the deeper it penetrates through the tissue. Scattering is defined by the laser energy that is directed away from the target. Light scattering decreases with increasing wavelength. Therefore, a laser with a low scattering coefficient makes a scalpel of the laser, while a high scattering coefficient results in a photocoagulator.

Examples of laser devices include long-pulsed lasers allow for slow heating of targets, and are effective for minimizing epidermal damage during laser hair removal. On the contrary, Q-switch lasers can deliver powerful, short pulses of light energy that shatter targets such as tattoo pigment in the dermis. Fractionated lasers (both non-ablative and ablative) create microscopic columns of coagulated or ablated tissue that are followed by re-epithelialization and dermal remodeling. Lastly, continuous and quasi-continuous lasers are no longer used often due to the increased risks of adverse effects secondary to excessive heating of tissue. An overview of the electromagnetic spectrum and medical laser wavelengths can be found in Figure 27. In all cases, appropriate pre-cautions should be taken as adverse health effects due to exposure to laser radiation are possible (wear specialized goggles, remove reflecting surfaces from the room like mirrors and jewelry, and attach laser-in-use signs to the entrance. The eye and skin are the most susceptible to damage by laser radiation. As with other tissues, the biological effects of laser on the eye vary depending upon the wavelength and exposure duration.[137]

Figure 28
Electromagnetic spectrum and medical laser wavelengths

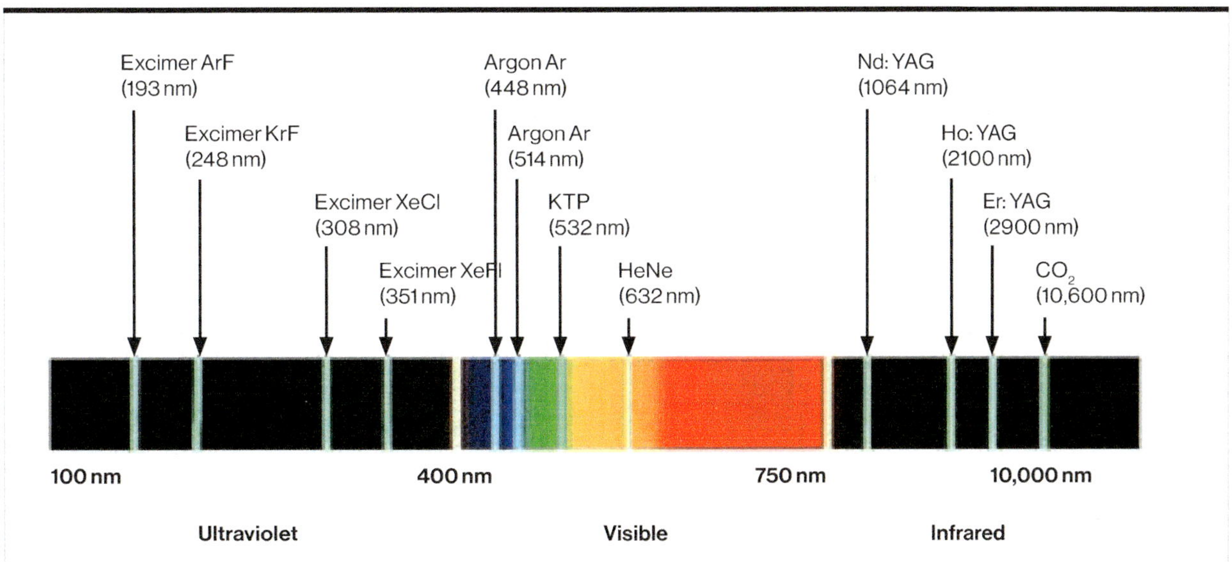

5.5 The future is here – special contributions

A novel Augmented Reality application for visualizing the patient's arteries

The vascular anatomy of the face is complex and above all extremely variable. Although profound anatomical knowledge is crucial to perform filler injections, it can also be argued that it's obsolete as the anatomy is so variable that the arteries are rarely where one would expect them. One of the most exciting inventions of the last decade, Augmented Reality, may potentially hold the solution to the difficult challenge to "see through someone's skin".

In search of a harmless method for the visualization of the individual arterial network of the face, a combined technique of infrared (IR) facial heating and Time of Flight magnetic resonance angiography (MRA) seems to be the preferred method.[177] Images are acquired on a 3 Tesla full-body MR system, using a dedicated head coil. Before the MRA examination, the patient's face is heated using an IR light source (300 W with an UV filter) for 10 minutes. This will induce vasodilata¬tion and enhance vascular flow. Using this protocol, a comprehensive overview of the facial arterial anatomy is created in a non-invasive way, without the use of intravenous contrast injections or radiation.[178]

The patented Artery3D technology (www.augmented-anatomy.com) processes the MRI images subsequently into an Augmented Reality image that is visualized using a smartphone. The process starts with extracting the intracranial vessels from the native MRI images, keeping only the subcutaneous arteries of the face, even with a diameter smaller than 1mm.[179] The vascular model is then converted into a 3D mesh that can be visualized through Augmented Reality (AR) using any smartphone. Hence, this technology allows anyone to see an individual's real and unique arterial anatomy in a dynamic way.

In recent clinical studies, the superficial temporal artery and supratrochlear artery were visualized in 100% of the patients, and the facial artery was visualized in 89% of the patients. The position of the visualized arteries was validated using Doppler Ultrasound, showing an average deviation of 0,3mm (SD +/- 0,7mm). The visualization of the perioral vessels, however, may be hindered by perioral artefacts and in patients with dental implants, fillings or dental wires after having had braces.[180, 205]
Looking at the future, the next step will be to get the ARtery3D technology ready for an AR-headset such as the HoloLens2 by Microsoft. This will allow the practitioner to keep both hands free and get a true 3D depth view of the anatomy.

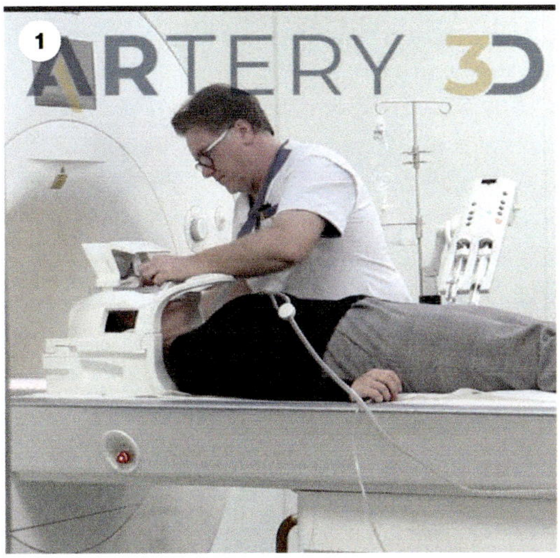

MRI of patient

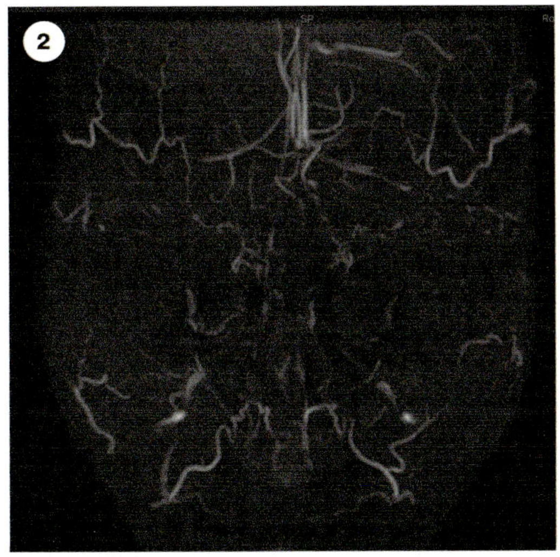

Uploaded to server

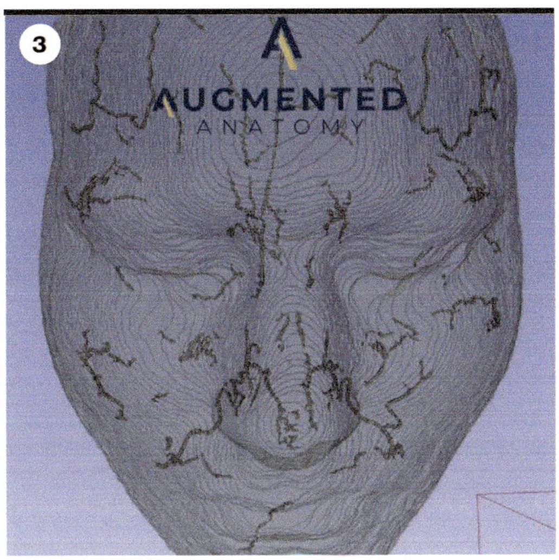

3D Augmented Reality version made

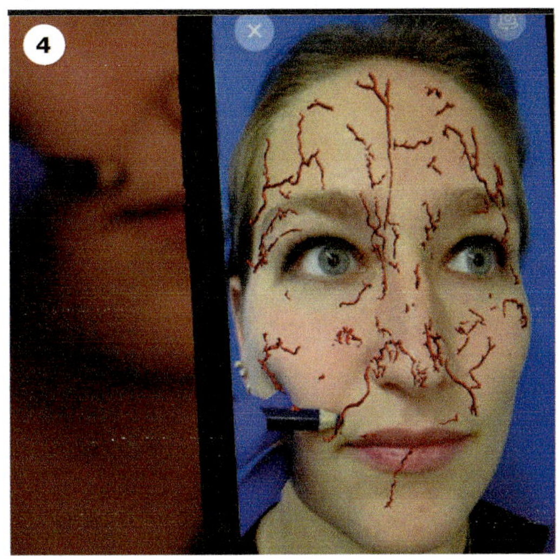

Arterial anatomy visible on smartphone

Figure 29
The different steps in making an augmented reality image of facial arterial structures using MRI.

1. f MRI of the patient;
2. MRI image is stored at the server;
3. The 3-D MRI of the arteries is matched with the uploaded 3-D scan of the patient's face.
4. Live inspection using iPhone visualizes the location of the patient's arteries in real time Augmented Reality.

DNA Filler test for detecting increased risk to late adverse events to soft tissue fillers

According to several scientific studies, in general there is a low risk of 1 to 3 out of 100 patients can have severe adverse events to soft tissue filler treatments.[88,169,181] Even though manufacturers claim that the soft tissue fillers are non-toxic and non-immunogenic, adverse events may occur. Clinically and histologically, most of the late onset adverse events present as an inflammatory response.[54,182] Most of these inflammatory responses seem to have an immunological basis, where the soft tissue fillers (=foreign body material) act as direct T-cell activators, on a possible background of genetic predisposition.[99] Furthermore, genes within the major histocompatibility complex (MHC) have been shown to play important roles in the development of a variety of autoimmune diseases in women with silicone breast implants.[183-184] Especially the HLA subtype-B*08 and HLA subtype-DRB1*03. After 6 years of research by the scientific team of the Vall d'Hebron University Hospital in Barcelona, Amsterdam UMC and Erasmus Medical Center in Rotterdam, they have found that there is a link between soft tissue fillers and adverse events for the patients in the study. For those people who had a combination of two specific genes, 84 out of 100 with this combination will have adverse events. Therefore, the DNA Filler test as offered through www.bsuremedical.com, detects if patients could be one of those who can have a higher change to adverse events to soft tissue filler treatments.

references

1. **American Society for Aesthetic Plastic Surgery (ASAPS).** *Cosmetic surgery national data bank statistics 2017.* http://www.surgery.org/sites/default/files/2014-Stats.pdf.: https://www.surgery.org/media/statistics. Consulted on August 5th, 2020.
2. **Lemperle G, Gauthier-Hazan N, Wolters M, et al.** *Foreign body granulomas after all injectable dermal fillers: Part 1. Possible causes. Plast Reconstr Surg.* 2008;123:1864–1873.
3. **van Loghem J, Humzah D, Kerscher M.** *Cannula Versus Sharp Needle for Placement of Soft Tissue Fillers: An Observational Cadaver Study* Aesthet Surg J. 2017 Dec 13;38(1):73-88
4. **Van Loghem JAJ, Siebenga PS, Thuis J.** *Vascular complications Part 1: Prevention.* PMFA. Oct /Nov 2020 | Vol 8 No 1.
5. **Van Loghem JAJ, Siebenga PS, Thuis J.** *Vascular complications part 2: management.* PMFA. DEC/JAN 2021 | Vol 8 No 2.
6. **Khan TT; Colon-Acevedo B, Mettu P, et al.** *An Anatomical Analysis of the Supratrochlear Artery: Considerations in Facial Filler Injections and Preventing Vision Loss.* Aesthetic Surgery Journal 20176, V1o–l637(2) 203–208.
7. **Saththianathan M, Johani K, Taylor A, et al.** *The Role of Bacterial Biofilm in Adverse Soft-Tissue Filler Reactions: A Combined Laboratory and Clinical Study.* Plast Reconstr Surg. 2017 Mar;139(3):613-621.
8. **Van Loghem JAJ, Fouché JJ, Thuis J.** *Sensitivity of aspiration as a safety test before injection of soft tissue fillers.* J Cosmet Dermatol. 2018 Feb;17(1):39-46.
9. **Sundaram H, Cassuto D.** *Biophysical characteristics of hyaluronic acid soft-tissue fillers and their relevance to aesthetic applications.* Plast Reconstr Surg. 2013;132(4 suppl 2):5S-21S.
10. **Sundaram H, Voigts B, Beer K, Meland M.** *Comparison of the rheo- logical properties of viscosity and elasticity in two categories of soft tissue fillers: calcium hydroxylapatite and hyaluronic acid.* Dermatol Surg. 2010;36:1859-1865.
11. **Elert G.** *"Viscosity". The physics hypertextbook.* (http://physics.info/ viscosity/). Retrieved December 2015–February 2016.
12. **King M.** *The management of bruising following nonsurgical cosmetic treatment.* J Clin Aesthet Dermatol. 2017;10:E1–E4.
13. **Gladstone HB, Cohen JL.** *Adverse effects when injecting facial fillers.* Semin Cutan Med Surg. 2007;26(1):34–39.
14. **Bailey SH, Cohen JL, Kenkel JM.** *Etiology, prevention, and treatment of dermal filler complications.* Aesthet Surg J. 2011;31(1):110–121.
15. **Fulton J, Caperton C, Weinkle S, Dewandre L.** *Filler injections with the blunt-tip microcannula.* J Drugs Dermatol. 2012;11(9):1098-1103.
16. **Zeichner JA, Cohen JL.** *Use of blunt tipped cannulas for soft tissue fillers.* J Drugs Dermatol. 2012;11(1):70–72.
17. **Signorini M, Liew S, Sundaram H, et al.** *Global Aesthetics Consensus: Avoidance and Management of Complications from Hyaluronic Acid Fillers-Evidence- and Opinion-Based Review and Consensus Recommendations.* Plast Reconstr Surg. 2016 Jun;137(6):961e-71e.
18. **Shah NS, Lazarus MC, Bugdodel R, et al.** *The effects of topical vitamin K on bruising after laser treatment.* J Am Acad Dermatol. 2002;47:241–244.
19. **Cohen JL, Bhatia AC.** *The role of topical vitamin K oxide gel in the resolution of postprocedural purpura.* J Drugs Dermatol. 2009;8:1020–1024.
20. **Snozzi P, van Loghem J.** *Complication Management following Rejuvenation Procedures with Hyaluronic Acid Fillers—an Algorithm-based Approach.* Plast Reconstr Surg Glob Open 2018;6:e2061.
21. **Funt D, Pavicic T.** *Dermal fillers in aesthetics: an overview of adverse events and treatment approaches.* Clin Cosmet Investig Dermatol. 2013 Dec 12;6:295-316.
22. **Toole BP.** *Hyaluronan: from extracellular glue to pericellular cue.* Nat Rev Cancer. 2004;4:528–539.
23. **Siebenga PS, van Amerongen G, Klaassen ES, et al.** *The ultraviolet B inflammation model: Postinflammatory hyperpigmentation and validation of a reduced UVB exposure paradigm for inducing hyperalgesia in healthy subjects.Eur* J Pain. 2019 May;23(5):874-883.
24. **Davis EC, Callender VD.** *Postinflammatory hyperpigmentation: A review of the epidemiology, clinical features, and treatment options in skin of color.* J Clin Aesthet Dermatol. 2010 Jul;3(7):20-31.
25. **Masu S, Seiji M.** *Pigmentary incontinence in fixed drug eruptions. Histologic and electron microscopic findings.* J Am Acad Dermatol. 1983 Apr;8(4):525-32.
26. **Taylor S, Grimes P, Lim J, et al.** *Postinflammatory hyperpigmentation.* J Cutan Med Surg. Jul-Aug 2009;13(4):183-91.
27. **Taylor SC, Burgess CM, Callender VD.** *Safety of nonanimal stabilized hyaluronic acid dermal fillers in patients with skin of color: a randomized, evaluator-blinded comparative trial.* Dermatol Surg. 2009;35:1653–1660.
28. **Heath CR, Taylor SC.** *Fillers in the skin of color population.* J Drugs Dermatol. 2011;10:494–498.
29. **Pavicic T.** *Efficacy and tolerability of a new monophasic, double- crosslinked hyaluronic acid filler for correction of deep lines and wrinkles.* J Drugs Dermatol. 2011;10(2):134-139.
30. **DeLorenzi C.** *Complications of injectable fillers, part I.* Aesthet Surg J. 2013;33:561–575.

31. **Orsini RA;** *Plastic Surgery Educational Foundation Technology Assessment Committee. Bromelain.* Plast Reconstr Surg. 2006;118:1640–1644.
32. **Abduljabbar MH, Basendwh MA.** *Complications of hyaluronic acid fillers and their managements.* J Dermatol Derm Surg. 2016;20:100–106.
33. **Yadav S, Dogra S.** *A cutaneous reaction to microneedling for postacne scarring caused by nickel hypersensitivity.* Aesthet Surg J. 2016;36:NP168–NP170.
34. **Geisler D, Shumer S, Elson ML.** *Delayed hypersensitivity reaction to Restylane®.* Cosmetic Dermatol. 2007;20(12):784–786.
35. **Arron ST, Neuhaus IM.** *Persistent delayed-type hypersensitivity reaction to injectable non-animal-stabilized hyaluronic acid.* J Cosmet Dermatol. 2007;6(3):167–171.
36. **Cassuto D, Marangoni O, De Santis G, Christensen L.** *Advanced laser techniques for filler-induced complications.* Dermatol Surg. 2009; 35 Suppl 2:1689–1695.
37. **Funt DK.** *Avoiding malar edema during midface/cheek augmentation with dermal fillers.* J Clin Aesthet Dermatol. 2011;4:32–36.
38. **Moffarah AS, Al Mohajer M, Hurwitz BL, Armstrong DG.** *Skin and Soft Tissue Infections.* Microbiol Spectr. 2016 Aug;4(4)
39. **Grice EA, Segre JA.** *The skin microbiome.* Nat Rev Microbiol. 2011 Apr;9(4):244-53.
40. **Ramakrishnan K, Salinas RC, Agudelo Higuita NI.** *Skin and Soft Tissue Infections.* Am Fam Physician. 2015 Sep 15;92(6):474-83.
41. **Eron LJ, Lipsky BA, Low DE, Nathwani D, Tice AD, Volturo GA,** *Expert panel on managing skin and soft tissue infections. Managing skin and soft tissue infections: expert panel recommendations on key decision points.* J Antimicrob Chemother . 2003 Nov;52 Suppl 1:i3-17.
42. **Olaniyi R, Pozzi C, Grimaldi L, Bagnoli F.** *Staphylococcus aureus-Associated Skin and Soft Tissue Infections: Anatomical Localization, Epidemiology, Therapy and Potential Prophylaxis.* Curr Top Microbiol Immunol. 2017;409:199-227.
43. **Stevens DL, Bisno AL, Chambers HF, Dellinger EP, Goldstein EJ, Gorbach SL, Hirschmann JV, Kaplan SL, Montoya JG, Wade JC; Infectious Diseases Society of America.** *Practice guidelines for the diagnosis and management of skin and soft tissue infections: 2014 update by the Infectious Diseases Society of America.* Clin Infect Dis. 2014 Jul 15;59(2):e10-52.
44. **Pasternack MS, Swartz MN.** *Cellulitis, necrotizing fasciitis, and subcutaneous tissue infections,* p. 1289–1312. In Mandell G, Bennet J, Dolin R (ed). Mandell, Douglas, and Bennett's Principles and Practice of Infectious Diseases. 2010. Elsevier, Philadelphia.
45. **Heydenrych I, Kapoor KM, De Boulle K, Goodman G, Swift A, Kumar N, Rahman E.** *A 10-point plan for avoiding hyaluronic acid dermal filler-related complications during facial aesthetic procedures and algorithms for management.* Clin Cosmet Investig Dermatol. 2018 Nov 23;11:603-611.
46. **Klastersky J.** *Infections in immunocompromised patients, I: pathogenesis, etiology, and diagnosis.* Clin Ther. 1985;8:90-99.
47. **Kadouch JA, Vos W, Nijhuis EW, Hoekzema R.** *Granulomatous foreign-body reactions to permanent fillers: detection of CD123+ plasmacytoid dendritic cells.* Am J Dermatopathol. 2015;37:107-114.
48. **Daley T, Damm DD, Haden JA, Kolodychak MT.** *Oral lesions associated with injected hydroxyapatite cosmetic filler. Oral Surg Oral Med Oral Pathol Oral Radiol.* 2012;114:107-111.
49. **Nicolau PJ.** *Long-lasting and permanent fillers: biomaterial influence over host tissue response.* Plast Reconstr Surg. 2007;119:2271-2286.
50. **Kadouch JA, Kadouch DJ, Fortuin S, van Rozelaar L, Karim RB, Hoekzema R.** *Delayed-onset complications of facial soft tissue augmentation with permanent fillers in 85 patients.* Dermatol Surg. 2013;39:1474-1485
51. **Graivier MH, Bass LM, Lorenc ZP, Fitzgerald R, Goldberg DJ, Lemperle G.** *Differentiating Nonpermanent Injectable Fillers: Prevention and Treatment of Filler Complications.* Aesthet Surg J. 2018 Apr 6;38(suppl_1):S29-S40.
52. **Paliwal S, Fagien S, Sun X, et al.** *Skin extracellular matrix stimulation following injection of a hyaluronic acid-based dermal filler in a rat model.* Plast Reconstr Surg. 2014;134:1224–1233.
53. **Lemperle G, Morhenn VB, Charrier U.** *Human histology and persistence of various injectable filler substances for soft tissue augmentation.* Aesthetic Plast Surg. 2003;27:354.
54. **Alijotas-Reig J, Fernández-Figueras MT, Puig L.** *Late-onset inflammatory adverse reactions related to soft tissue filler injections.* Clin Rev Allergy Immunol. 2013;45(1):97–108.
55. **Rayahin JE, Buhrman JS, Zhang Y, et al.** *High and low molecular weight hyaluronic acid differentially influence macrophage activation.* ACS Biomater Sci Eng. 2015;1:481–493.
56. **Schelke LW, Decates TS, van der Lugt CIM, et al.** *Intralesional laser treatment for dermal filler complications.* Plast Reconstr Surg. 2018;141:1361–1369.
57. **Christensen LH.** *Host tissue interaction, fate, and risks of degradable and nondegradable gel fillers.* Dermatol Surg. 2009;35 Suppl 2: 1612–1619.
58. **Monheit GD, Rohrich RJ.** *The nature of long-term fillers and the risk of complications.* Dermatol Surg. 2009;35 Suppl 2:1598–1604.

references

59. **Hanke CW, Redbord KP.** *Safety and efficacy of poly-L-lactic acid in HIV lipoatrophy and lipoatrophy of aging.* J Drugs Dermatol. 2007;6(2):123-128.
60. **Kadouch JA.** *Calcium hydroxylapatite: a review on safety and complications.* J Cosmet Dermatol. 2017;16(2):152-161.
61. **Rayess HM, Svider PF, Hanba C, et al.** *A cross-sectional analysis of adverse events and litigation for injectable fillers.* JAMA Facial Plast Surg. 2018;20(3):207-214.
62. **Van Loghem JAJ, Funt D, Pavicic T, et al.** *Managing intravascular complications following treatment with calcium hydroxylapatite: An expert consensus.* J Cosmet Dermatol. 2020;00:1–14.
63. **DeLorenzi C.** *Transarterial degradation of HA filler by hyaluronidase.* Dermatol Surg. 2014;40(8):832–841.
64. **Cohen JL, Biesman BS, Dayan SH, DeLorenzi C, Lambros VS, Nestor MS, Sadick N, Sykes J.** *Treatment of hyaluronic acid filler-Iinduced impending necrosis with hyaluronidase: consensus recommendations.* Aesthet Surg J. 2015;35(7):844-849.
65. **King M, Convery C, Davies E.** *The use of hyaluronidase in aesthetic practice.* J Clin Aesthet Dermatol 2018;11(6):428-434.
66. **DeLorenzi C.** *New high dose pulsed hyaluronidase protocol for hyaluronic acid filler vascular adverse events.* Aesthetic Surg J. 2017;37:1–12.
67. **Dayan SH, Arkins JP, Mathison CC.** *Management of impending necrosis associated with soft tissue filler injections.* J Drugs Dermatol 2011 Sep;10(9):1007-12.
68. **Loh KT, Chua JJ, Lee HM, et al.** *Prevention and management of vision loss relating to facial filler injections.* Singapore Med J. 2016;57:438–443.
69. **Carruthers J, Fagien S, Dolman P.** *Retro or PeriBulbar injection techniques to reverse visual loss after filler injections.* Dermatol Surg. 2015;41:S354–S357.
70. **Carruthers JD, Fagien S, Rohrich RJ, et al.** *Blindness caused by cosmetic filler injection: a review of cause and therapy.* Plast Reconstr Surg. 2014;134:1197–1201.
71. **International Society of Aesthetic Plastic Surgery (ISAPS).** *ISAPS international survey on aesthetic/cosmetic procedures performed in 2017.* https://www.isaps.org/wp-content/uploads/2019/03/ ISAPS_2017_International_Study_Cosmetic_Procedures_NEW.pdf. Accessed May 19, 2019.
72. **Ashton MW, Taylor GI, Corlett RJ** *The Role of Anastomotic Vessels in Controlling Tissue Viability and Defining Tissue Necrosis with Special Reference to Complications following Injection of Hyaluronic Acid Fillers.* Reconstr Surg. 2018 Jun;141(6):818e-830e.
73. **DeLorenzi C.** *Complications of injectable fillers, part 2: vascular complications.* Aesthet Surg J. 2014;34:584–600.
74. **Von Arx T, Tamura K, Yukiya O, et al.** *The Face – A Vascular Perspective. A literature review.* Swiss Dent J. 2018 May 14;128(5):382-392.
75. **Chang S, Yousefi S, Qin J, et al.** *External compression versus intravascular injection: A mechanistic animal model of filler-induced tissue ischemia.* Ophthal Plast Reconstr Surg. 2016;32(4):261-266.
76. **Beleznay K , Carruthers JD , Humphrey S, et al.** *Avoiding and Treating Blindness From Fillers: A Recent Review of the World Literature.* Dermatol Surg. 2015 Oct;41(10):1097-117.
77. **Beleznay K , Carruthers JD , Humphrey S, et al.** *Update on Avoiding and Treating Blindness From Fillers: A Recent Review of the World Literature.* Aesthet Surg J. 2019 May 16;39(6):662-674.
78. **Lazzeri D, Agostini T, Figus M, et al.** *Blindness following cosmetic injections of the face.* Plast Reconstr Surg. 2012;129:995–1012.
79. **Thanasarnaksorn W, Cotofana S, Rudolph C, Kraisak P, Chanasumon N, Suwanchinda A.** *Severe vision loss caused by cosmetic filler aug- mentation: case series with review of cause and therapy.* J Cosmet Dermatol. 2018;17(5):712-718.
80. **Baker DL.** *Gentle, prolonged ocular massage can restore vision after retinal artery occlusion.* Healio.com website. Ocular Surgery News U.S. https://www.healio.com/news/ophthalmology/20120331/gentle-prolonged-ocular-massage-can-restore-vision-after-retinal-artery-occlusion. Edition. July 1, 2004. Accessed July 26th, 2020.
81. **Walker L, King M.** *This month's guideline: visual loss secondary to cosmetic filler injection.* J Clin Aesthet Dermatol. 2018;11(5):E53-E55.
82. **Schelke LW, Velthuis PJ, Kadouch J, Swift A.** *Early ultrasound for diagnosis and treatment of vascular adverse events with hyaluronic acid fillers.* J Am Acad Dermatol. 2019 Jul 17;S0190-9622(19)32392-8.
83. **Roberts SA, Arthurs BP.** *Severe visual loss and orbital infarction following periorbital aesthetic poly-(L)-lactic acid (PLLA) injection.* Ophthalmic Plast Reconstr Surg. May-Jun 2012;28(3):e68-70.
84. **Altintas H, Odemis M, Bilgi S, et al.** *Long-term complications of polyethylene glycol injection to the face.* Aesthetic Plast Surg 2012;36:427–30.
85. **De Vries C, Geertsma R.** *Clinical data on injectable tissue fillers: a review. Expert Rev. Med. Devices* 10(6), 835–853 (2013).
86. **Ramires PA, Miccoli MA, Panzarini L, et al.** *In vitro and in vivo biocompatibility of a polyalkylimide hydrogel for soft tissue augmentation.* J of Biomed Materials Research. 2005;72:230e8

87. **Protopapa C, Sito G, Caporale, et al.** *Bio-alcamid in drug- induced lipodystrophy.* J Cosmetic & Laser Ther 2003;5:226e30.
88. **Nelson L, Steward KJ.** *Early and late complications of polyalkylimide gel (Bio-Alcamid)®.* Journal of Plastic, Reconstructive & Aesthetic Surgery (2011) 64, 401-405.
89. **Christensen LH, Breiting VB, Aasted A, Jørgensen A, Kebuladze I.** *Long-term effects of polyacrylamide hydrogel on human breast tissue.* Plast Reconstr Surg. 2003;111(6):1883–1890.
90. **Yamauchi PS.** *Emerging permanent filler technologies: focus on Aquamid.* Clinical, Cosmetic and Investigational Dermatology 2014:7 261–266.
91. **Fernández-Cossío S, Castaño-Oreja MT.** *Biocompatibility of two novel dermal fillers: histological evaluation of implants of a hyaluronic acid filler and a polyacrylamide filler.* Plast Reconstr Surg. 2006;117(6): 1789–1796.
92. **Brooks N.** *A foreign body granuloma produced by an injectable collagen implant at a test site.* J Dermatol Surg Oncol. 1982;8:111.
93. **Rapaport MJ,Vinnik C,Zarem H.** *Injectable silicone: Cause of facial nodules, cellulites, ulceration, and migration.* Aesthetic Plast Surg. 1996;20:267.
94. **Duffy DM.** *Liquid silicone for soft tissue augmentation: Histological, clinical, and molecular perspectives.* Dermatol Surg. 2007;31:1530.
95. **Hexsel DM, Hexsel CL, Iyengar V.** *Liquid injectable silicone: History, mechanism of action, indications, technique, and complications.* Semin Cutan Med Surg. 2003;22:107.
96. **Senet P, Bachelez H, Ollivaud L, et al.** *Minocycline for the treatment of cutaneous silicone granulomas.* Br J Dermatol. 1999;140:985.
97. **Bigata X, Ribera M, Bielsa I, et al.** *Adverse granulomatous reaction after cosmetic dermal silicone injection.* Dermatol Surg. 2001;27:198.
98. **Requena L, Requena C, Christensen L, et al.** *Adverse reactions to injectable soft tissue fillers.* J Am Acad Dermatol. 2011;64:1.
99. **Alijotas-Reig J, Fernández-Figueras MT, Puig L.** *Inflammatory, immun–mediated adverse reactions related to soft tissue dermal fillers.* Semin Arthritis Rheum. 2013;43(2):241-58.
100. **Daines SM, Williams EF.** *Complications associated with injectable soft- tissue fillers: a 5-year retrospective review.* JAMA Facial Plast Surg. 2013;15:226.
101. **Zimmermann US, Clerici TJ.** *The histological aspects of filler complications.* Semin Cutan Med Surg. 2004;23:241.
102. **Christensen L, Breiting V, Janssen M, et al.** *Adverse reactions to injectable soft tissue permanent fillers.* Aesthet Plast Surg. 2005;29:34.
103. **Parada MB, Michalany NS, Hassun KM, et al.** *A histologic study of adverse effects of different cosmetic skin fillers. Skinmed. 2005;4:345. 21. Christensen L. Normal and pathologic tissue reactions to soft tissue gel fillers.* Dermatol Surg. 2007;33:S168.
104. **Dadzie OE, Mahalingam M, Parada M, et al.** *Adverse cutaneous reactions to soft tissue fillers—a review of the histological features.* J Cutan Pathol. 2008;35:536.
105. **Ledon JA, Savas JA, Yang S, et al.** *Inflammatory nodules following soft tissue filler use: a review of causative agents, pathology and treatment options.* Am J Clin Dermatol. 2013;14:401–411.
106. **Gelfer A, Carruthers A, Carruthers J, et al.** *The natural history of polymethylmethacrylate microspheres granulomas.* Dermatol Surg 2007;33:614–20.
107. **Kunjur J, Whiterow H.** *Long-term complications associated with permanent dermal fillers.* British Journal of Oral and Maxillofacial Surgery 51 (2013) 858–862.
108. **Rohrich RJ, Monheit G, Nguyen AT, et al.** *Soft–tissue filler com- plications: the important role of biofilms.* Plast Reconstr Surg 2010;125:1250–6 [Erratum in: Plast Reconstr Surg 2010;125:1850].
109. **Zeng M, Zhi-Yong L, Ma J, et al.** *Clarithromycin and dexamethasone show similar anti-inflammatory effects on distinct phenotypic chronic rhinosinusitis: An explant model study.* BMC Immunol. 2015;16:37.
110. **Nozoe K, Aida Y, Fukuda T, Sanui T, Nishimura F.** *Mechanisms of the macrolide-induced inhibition of superoxide generation by neutrophils. Inflammation* 2016;39:1039–1048.
111. **Cassuto D, Pignatti M, Pacchioni L, Boscaini G, Spaggiari A, De Santis G.** *Management of complications caused by permanent fillers in the face: A treatment algorithm.* Plast Reconstr Surg. 2016;138:215e–227e.
112. **Buhren BA, Schrumpf H, Hoff NP, et al.** *Hyaluronidase: from clinical applications to molecular and cellular mechanisms.* Eur J Med 19. Res. 2016;21:5.
113. **King M, Convery C, Davies E.** *The Use of Hyaluronidase in Aesthetic Practice (v2.4).* J Clin Aesthet Dermatol. 2018 Jun;11(6):E61-E68.
114. **Quezada-Gaón N, Wortsman X.** *Ultrasound-guided hyaluronidase injection in cosmetic complications.* J Eur Acad Dermatol Venereol. 2016;30(10):e39–e40. 23.
115. **Bailey SH, Fagien S, Rohrich RJ.** *Changing role of hyaluronidase in plastic surgery.* Plast Reconstr Surg. 2014;133(2):127e-132e.
116. **Papakonstantinou E, Roth M, Karakiulakis G.** *HA: A key molecule in skin aging. Dermatoendocrinol.* 2012;4(3):253–258.

references

117. **Meyer K.** *Hyaluronidases. In: Boyer PD, ed. The Enzymes. New York,* NY: Academic Press (1971):307–320.

118. **Bell L, McAdams T, Morgan R, Parshley PF, Pike RC, Riggs P, et al.** *Pruritus in burns: a descriptive study.* J Burn Care Rehabil 1988;9:305-8.

119. **Bayat A, McGrouther DA, Ferguson MWJ.** *Skin scarring.* BMJ. 2003 Jan 11;326(7380):88-92.

120. **Niessen FB, Spauwen PH, Schalkwijk J, Kon M.** *On the nature of hyper- trophic scars and keloids: a review.* Plast Reconstr Surg 1999;104:1435-58.

121. **Van den Helder CJ, Hage JJ.** *Sense and nonsense of scar creams and gels.* Aesthetic Plast Surg 1994;18:307-13.

122. **Uppal RS, Khan U, Kakar S, Talas G, Chapman P, McGrouther DA.** *The effects of a single dose of 5-fluorouracil on keloid scars: a clinical trial of timed wound irrigation after extralesional excision.* Plast Reconstr Surg 2001;108:1218-24.

123. **Broker BJ, Rosen D, Amsberry J, Schmidt R, Sailor L, Pribitkin EA, et al.** *Keloid excision and recurrence prophylaxis via intradermal interferon- gamma injections: a pilot study.* Laryngoscope 1996;106(12 Pt 1):1497- 501.

124. **Espana A ,Solano T, Quintanilla E.** *Bleomycinin the treatment of keloids and hypertrophic scars by multiple needle punctures.* Dermatol Surg 2001;27:23-7.

125. **Clavere P, Bedane C, Bonnetblanc JM, Bonnafoux-Clavere A, Rousseau J.** *Postoperative interstitial radiotherapy of keloids by iridium 192: a retrospective study of 46 treated scars.* Dermatology 1997;195:349-52.

126. **Alster TS, Williams CM.** *Treatment of keloid sternotomy scars with 585 nm flashlamp-pumped pulsed-dye laser.* Lancet 1995;345:1198-200.

127. **Zouboulis CC, Zouridaki E, Rosenberger A, Dalkowski A.** *Current developments and uses of cryosurgery in the treatment of keloids and hyper- trophic scars.* Wound Repair Regen 2002;10:98-102.

128. **Hirsch RJ, Lewis AB.** *Treatment of acne scarring.* Semin Cutan Med Surg 2001;20:190-8.

129. **Jordan RB, Daher J, Wasil K.** *Splints and scar management for acute and reconstructive burn care.* Clin Plast Surg 2000;27:71-85.

130. **Darzi MA, Chowdri NA, Kaul SK, Khan M.** *Evaluation of various methods of treating keloids and hypertrophic scars: a 10-year follow-up study.* Br J Plast Surg 1992;45:374-9.

131. **Urioste SS, Arndt KA, Dover JS.** *Keloids and hypertrophic scars: review and treatment strategies.* Semin Cutan Med Surg 1999;18:159-71.

132. **Adant JP, Bluth F, Jacquemin D.** *Reconstruction of neck burns. A long-term comparative study between skin grafts, skin expansion and free flaps.* Acta Chir Belg 1998;98:5-9.

133. **Soliman YS, Horowitz R, Hashim PW.** *Update on Acne Scar Treatment. Cutis.* 2018;102:21-25, 47-48.

134. **You H, Kim D, Yoon E, et al.** *Comparison of four different lasers for acne scars: resurfacing and fractional lasers.* J Plast Reconstr Aesthet Surg. 2016;69:E87-E95.

135. **Anderson RR, Parrish JA.** *Selective photothermolysis: precise microsurgery by selective absorption of pulsed radiation.* Science 1983; 220:524.

136. **Polanyi TG.** *Physics of surgery with lasers.* Clin Chest Med 1985; 6:179.

137. **Occupational Safety and Health Administration.** www.osha.gov.

138. **Yutskovskaya and Kogan.** *Improved Neocollagenesis and Skin Mechanical Properties After Injection of Diluted Calcium Hydroxylapatite in the Neck and Décolletage: A Pilot Study,* J Drugs Dermatol. 2017;16(1):68-74.

139. **Vrcek IM, Malouf P, Gilliland DG.** *A Novel Solution for Superficially Placed Calcium Hydroxylapatite (Radiesse) in the Inferior Eyelid.* Orbit, 31(6), 431–432, 2012

140. **Kavitha K et al.** *Calcium Hydroxylapatite Nodule Resolution After Fractional Carbon Dioxide Laser Therapy.* Arch Dermatol. 2012;148(5):634-636

141. **Shalmon D, Cohen JL, Landau M et al.** *Management Patterns of Delayed Inflammatory Reactions to Hyaluronic Acid Dermal Fillers: An Online Survey in Israel.* Clin Cosmet Investig Dermatol. 2020 May 7;13:345-349.

142. **Artzi O, Cohen JL, Dover JS, et al.** *Delayed Inflammatory Reactions to Hyaluronic Acid Fillers: A Literature Review and Proposed Treatment Algorithm.* Clin Cosmet Investig Dermatol. 2020 May 18;13:371-378.

143. **Madoff SE, Urquiaga M, Alonso CD, Kelly CP.** *Prevention of recurrent Clostridioides difficile infection: a systematic review of randomized controlled trials.* Anaerobe. 2020;61:102098.

144. **Aguilera SB, Ariztizabal M, Reed A.** *Successful Treatment of Calcium Hydroxylapatite Nodules With Intralesional 5-Fluorouracil, Dexamethasone, and Triamcinolone.* J Drugs Dermatol. 2016 Sep 1;15(9):1142-3.

145. **Saari H, Konttinen YT, Friman C, Sorsa T.** *Differential effects of reactive oxygen species on native synovial fluid and purified human umbilical cord hyaluronate".* Inflammation 1993. 17 (4): 403–15.

146. **Lemperle G, Gaulthier-Hazan N.** *Foreign body granulomas after all injectable dermal fillers. Part 2 Treatment options.* Plast Reconstr Surg. 2008:123.1864-1873

147. **Vleggaar D, Fitzgerald R, et al.** *Consensus recommendations on the use of injectable poly-L-lactic acid for facial and nonfacial volumization.* J Drugs Dermatol. 2014 Apr;13(4 Suppl):s44-51.

148. **Anderson JM, Rodriguez A, Chang DT.** *Foreign body*

reaction to biomaterials. Semin Immunol. 2008;20(2):86-100.

149. **Lowe NJ, Maxwell CA, Patnaik R.** *Adverse reactions to dermal fillers: review.* Dermatol Surg. 2005;31(11 Pt 2):1616-25.
150. **Duranti F, Salti G, Bovani B, Calandra M, Rosati ML.** *Injectable hyaluronic acid gel for soft tissue augmentation. A clinical and histological study.* Dermatol Surg. 1998;24(12):1317-25.
151. **Lombardi T, Samson J, Plantier F, Husson C, Kuffer R.** *Orofacial granulomas after injection of cosmetic fillers. Histopathologic and clinical study of 11 cases.* J Oral Pathol Med. 2004;33(2):115-20.
152. **Mariani E, Lisignoli G, Borzi RM, Pulsatelli L.** *Biomaterials: Foreign Bodies or Tuners for the Immune Response?* Int J Mol Sci. 2019;20(3).
153. **Christensen L, Breiting V, Bjarnsholt T, Eickhardt S, Hogdall E, Janssen M, et al.** *Bacterial infection as a likely cause of adverse reactions to polyacrylamide hydrogel fillers in cosmetic surgery.* Clin Infect Dis. 2013;56(10):1438-44.
154. **Lemperle G, Rullan PP, Gauthier-Hazan N.** *Avoiding and treating dermal filler complications.* Plast Reconstr Surg. 2006;118(3 Suppl):92S-107S.
155. **Orentreich DS.** *Liquid injectable silicone: techniques for soft tissue augmentation.* Clin Plast Surg. 2000;27(4):595-612.
156. **Rongioletti F, Cattarini G, Sottofattori E, Rebora A.** *Granulomatous reaction after intradermal injections of hyaluronic acid gel.* Arch Dermatol. 2003;139(6):815-6.
157. **Alhede M, Er O, Eickhardt S, Kragh K, Alhede M, Christensen LD, et al.** *Bacterial biofilm formation and treatment in soft tissue fillers.* Pathog Dis. 2014;70(3):339-46.
158. **Lemperle G, Nicolau P, Scheiermann N.** *Is there any evidence for biofilms in dermal fillers?* Plast Reconstr Surg. 2011;128(2):84e-5e.
159. **Morhenn VB, Lemperle G, Gallo RL.** *Phagocytosis of different particulate dermal filler substances by human macrophages and skin cells.* Dermatol Surg. 2002;28(6):484-90.
160. **Lemperle G, Morhenn VB, Pestonjamasp V, Gallo RL.** *Migration studies and histology of injectable microspheres of different sizes in mice.* Plast Reconstr Surg. 2004;113(5):1380-90.
161. **Tomazic-Jezic VJ, Merritt K, Umbreit TH.** *Significance of the type and the size of biomaterial particles on phagocytosis and tissue distribution.* J Biomed Mater Res. 2001;55(4):523-9.
162. **Bergeret-Galley C, Latouche X, Illouz YG.** *The value of a new filler material in corrective and cosmetic surgery: DermaLive and DermaDeep.* Aesthetic Plast Surg. 2001;25(4):249-55.
163. **Eppley BL, Summerlin DJ, Prevel CD, Sadove AM.** *Effects of a positively charged biomaterial for dermal and subcutaneous augmentation.* Aesthetic Plast Surg. 1994;18(4):413-6.
164. **Misiek DJ, Kent JN, Carr RF.** *Soft tissue responses to hydroxylapatite particles of different shapes.* J Oral Maxillofac Surg. 1984;42(3):150-60.
165. **Taylor SR, Gibbons DF.** *Effect of surface texture on the soft tissue response to polymer implants.* J Biomed Mater Res. 1983;17(2):205-27.
166. **Brahm J, Lessel R, Ditlev S, Schmidt R, editors.** *Determination of water and solute transport in polyacrylamide gels.* Macromolecular symposia; 2008: Wiley Online Library.
167. **Keen MA.** *Hyaluronic Acid in Dermatology.* Skinmed. 2017;15(6):441-8.
168. **Kim JE, Sykes JM.** *Hyaluronic acid fillers: history and overview.* Facial Plast Surg. 2011;27(6):523-8.
169. **Artzi O, Loizides C, Verner I, Landau M.** *Resistant and Recurrent Late Reaction to Hyaluronic Acid-Based Gel.* Dermatol Surg. 2016 Jan;42(1):31-7. doi: 10.1097/DSS.0000000000000562. PMID: 26655699.
170. **Marusza W, Olszanski R, Sierdzinski J, Ostrowski T, Szyller K, Mlynarczyk G, et al.** *Treatment of late bacterial infections resulting from soft-tissue filler injections.* Infect Drug Resist. 2019;12:469-80.
171. **Beleznay K, Carruthers JD, Carruthers A, Mummert ME, Humphrey S.** *Delayed-onset nodules secondary to a smooth cohesive 20 mg/mL hyaluronic acid filler: cause and management.* Dermatol Surg. 2015;41(8):929-39.
172. **Broly M, Marie J, et al.** Management of granulomatous foreign body reaction to fillers with methotrexate. JEADV 2020;34(4):817-820.
173. **Munavali GG, Guthridge R, et al.** *"COVID-19/SARS-CoV-2 virus spike protein-related delayed inflammatory reaction to hyaluronic acid dermal fillers: a challenging clinical conundrum in diagnosis and treatment"*
174. **Munavali GG, Knutsen Larsson S, et al.** *Oral angiotensin-converting enzyme inhibitors for treatment of delayed inflammatory reaction to dermal hyaluronic acid fillers following COVID-19 vaccination-a model for inhibition of angiotensin II-induced cutaneous inflammation.* JAAD Case Reports 2021;10:63-8.
175. **IM. Vrcek et. al.** *A Novel Solution for Superficially Placed Calcium Hydroxylapatite (Radiesse) in the Inferior Eyelid. Orbit,* 2012;31(6):431–432
176. **K. Kavitha et al.** *Calcium Hydroxylapatite Nodule*

references

Resolution After Fractional Carbon Dioxide Laser Therapy. Arch Dermatol. 2012;148(5):634-636.

177. **Cavallini M, Trocchi G, Heyndrich I, De Boulle K, Hendrickx B, Pirayeshi A.** *Complications of absorbable fillers, In 'Aesthetic facial anatomy essentials for injections'* by CRC Press 2020, ISBN 9781138505728
178. **Hendrickx B, Waked K, Mespreuve M.** *Infrared Thermally Enhanced 3-Dimensional Time of Flight Magnetic Resonance Angiography Imaging for the Visualization of the Arteries of the Face.* Aesthetic surgery journal open forum 2020, 1–10
179. **Mespreuve M, Waked K, Hendrickx B.** *Visualization techniques of the facial arteries.* J cosmet dermatol 2020 may 27.doi: 10.1111
180. **Mespreuve M, Waked K, Hendrickx B.** *The usefulness of Magnetic Resonance Angiography to analyse the variable arterial facial anatomy in an effort to reduce filler-associated blindness: anatomical study and visualisation through an augmented reality application.* Aesthetic Surgery Journal Open Forum 2021, Accepted for publication.
181. **Karim RB, Hage JJ, van Rozelaar L, Lange CA, Raaijmakers J.** *Complications of polyalkylimide 4% injections (Bio-Alcamid): a report of 18 cases.* J Plast Reconstr Aesthet Surg 2006;59:1409-14.
182. **Alijotas-Reig J, Garcia-Gimenez V, Miró-Mur F, Vilardell-Tarrés M.** *Delayed immune-mediated adverse effects of polyalkylimide dermal fillers: clinical findings and long-term follow-up.* Arch Dermatol 2008;144(5):637-42. Erratum in: Arch Dermatol 2008;144(8):1082.
183. **Moling O, Piccin A, Tauber M, et al.** *Intravascular large B-cell lymphoma associated with silicone breast implant, HLA-DRB1*11:01, and HLA-DQB1*03:01 manifesting as macrophage activation syndrome and with severe neurological symptoms: a case report.* J Med Case Rep 2016 Sep 15;10(1):254.
184. **Di Lorenzo G, Mansueto P, Melluso M, et al.** *Morphea after silicone gel breast implantation for cosmetic reasons in an HLA-B8, DR3-positive woman.* Int Arch Allergy Immunol 1997 Jan;112(1):93-5.
185. **Brown SA, Rorich R, Baumann, L et al.** *Subject global evaluation and subject satisfaction using injectable poly-L-lactic acid versus human collagen for the correction of nasolabial fold wrinkles.* Plastic & Reconstructive Surgery 2011, 127(4) 1684-1692
186. **Fitzgerald R and Vleggaar D.** *Facial volume restoration of the aging face with poly-l-lactic acid.* Dermatol.Ther. 2011; 24 2-27
187. **Kadouch JA, Vos W, Nijhuis EWP and Hoekzema R.** *Granulomatous foreign-body reactions to permanent fillers: detection of CD123+ plasmacytoid dendritic cells.* Am J Dermatopathol. 2015 Feb;37(2):107-14.
188. **Decates TS, Velthuis PJ, Schelke LW, et al.** *Increased risk of late-onset, immune-mediated, adverse reactions related to dermal fillers in patients bearing HLA-B*08 and DRB1*03 haplotypes.* Dermatol Ther. 2021 Jan;34(1):e14644.
189. **Taylor GI, Chubb DP, Ashton MW.** *True and 'choke' anastomoses between perforator angiosomes: part i. anatomical location.* Plast Reconstr Surg. 2013 Dec;132(6):1447-1456.
190. **Jajoria H, Venkataram A, Mysore V.** *Importance of Choke Vessels in Injectable Fillers.* J Cutan Aesthet Surg. Jul-Sep 2020;13(3):185-190.
191. **Brodmann M.** *The angiosome concept in clinical Practice. Implications for patient-specific recanalization procedures.* J Cardiovasc Surg (Torino). 2013 Oct;54(5):567-71.
192. **Qing L, Lei P, Tang J, et al.** *Inflammatory response associated with choke vessel remodeling in the extended perforator flap model.* Exp Ther Med. 2017 May;13(5):2012-2018.
193. **King M, Walker L, Convery C, Davies E.** *Management of a Vascular Occlusion Associated with Cosmetic Injections.* J Clin Aesthet Dermatol. 2020 Jan;13(1):E53-E58. Epub 2020 Jan 1.
194. **Wibowo A, Kapoor KM, Philipp-Dormston WG.** *Reversal of Post-filler Vision Loss and Skin Ischaemia with High-Dose Pulsed Hyaluronidase Injections.* Aesth Plast Surg43, 1337–1344 (2019).
195. **Chesnut, Cameron MD** *Restoration of Visual Loss With Retrobulbar Hyaluronidase Injection After Hyaluronic Acid Filler,* Dermatologic Surgery: March 2018 - Volume 44 - Issue 3 - p 435-437 doi: 10.1097/ DSS.0000000000001237
196. **Guo-Zhang Z, Zhong-Sheng S, Wen-Xiong L, et al.** *Efficacy of Retrobulbar Hyaluronidase Injection for Vision Loss Resulting from Hyaluronic Acid Filler Embolization,* Aesthetic Surgery Journal, Volume 38, Issue 1, January 2018, Pages 12–22.
197. **Zhang L, Pan L, Xu H. et al. (2019).** *Clinical Observations and the Anatomical Basis of Blindness After Facial Hyaluronic Acid Injection.* Aesthetic plastic surgery, 43(4), 1054–1060.
198. **Adulkar N, Cheng C, Lee, et al. (2019).** *An In Vitro Model Assessing the Penetration of Hyaluronidase through Optic Nerve Dura for Management of Hyaluronic Acid Facial Filler Embolism.* Plastic and reconstructive surgery, 144(1), 43e–47e.
199. **Lee W, Oh W, Ko HS, et al. (2019).** *Effectiveness of Retrobulbar Hyaluronidase Injection in an Iatrogenic*

Blindness Rabbit Model Using Hyaluronic Acid Filler Injection. Plastic and reconstructive surgery, 144(1), 137–143.

200. De Schaepdrijver L, Simoens P, Lauwers H, De Geest JP. (1989). *Retinal vascular patterns in domestic animals.* Research in veterinary science, 47(1), 34–42.

201. Hayreh SS, Zimmerman B, Kimura A, Sanon A. *Central retinal artery occlusion.: Retinal survival time, Experimental Eye Research,* Volume 78, Issue 3, 2004, Pages 723-736.

202. Tobalem S, Schutz JS, Chronopoulos A. (2018). *Central retinal artery occlusion - rethinking retinal survival time.* BMC ophthalmology, 18(1), 101.

203. Gutierrez P, Riveros P. (2021). *Retrobulbar Block. In StatPearls.* StatPearls Publishing.

204. Fahmi A, Bowman R. *Administering an eye anaesthetic: principles, techniques, and complications.* Community Eye Health. 2008 Mar;21(65):14-7.

205. Waked K, Mespreuve M, De Ranter J, Collard B, Hahn S, Hendrickx B. *Visualizing the Individual Arterial Anatomy of the Face Through Augmented Reality - A Useful and Accurate Tool During Dermal Filler Injections.* Aesthet Surg J Open Forum 2022.

206. Bachour Y, Bekkenk MW, Rustemeyer T, Kadouch JA. *Late inflammatory reactions in patients with soft tissue fillers after SARS-CoV-2 infection and vaccination: A systematic review of the literature.* J Cosmet Dermatol. 2022 Apr;21(4):1361-1368.

207. Munavalli GG, Guthridge R, Knutsen-Larson S, Brodsky A, Matthew E, Landau M. *COVID-19/SARS-CoV-2 virus spike protein-related delayed inflammatory reaction to hyaluronic acid dermal fillers: a challenging clinical conundrum in diagnosis and treatment.* Arch Dermatol Res. 2022 Jan;314(1):1-15.

208. Bentkover SH: *The biology of facial fillers.* Facial Plast Surg 2009; 25: 73–85

209. Fischer J, Metzler G, Schaller M. *Cosmetic permanent fillers for soft tissue augmentation: a new contraindication for interferon therapies.* Arch Dermatol. 2007; 143: 507–510

210. Bjarnsholt T et al.: *Detection of bacteria by fluorescence in situ hybridization in culture-negative soft tissue filler lesions.* Dermatol Surg. 2009; 35(Suppl 2): 1620-4

211. Alhede M et al.: *Bacterial biofilm formation and treatment in soft tissue fillers.* Pathog Dis 2014; 70: 339-46

212. Nygart JF et al.: *Effect of prophylactic antibiotics on polyacrylamide gel safety in facial augmentation.* J Drugs Dermatol 2014; 13(5): 571-3

213. Bachour Y, Bekkenk MW, Rustemeyer T, Kadouch JA. *Late inflammatory reactions in patients with soft tissue fillers after SARS-CoV-2 infection and vaccination: A systematic review of the literature.* J Cosmet Dermatol. 2022 Apr; 21(4):1361-1368

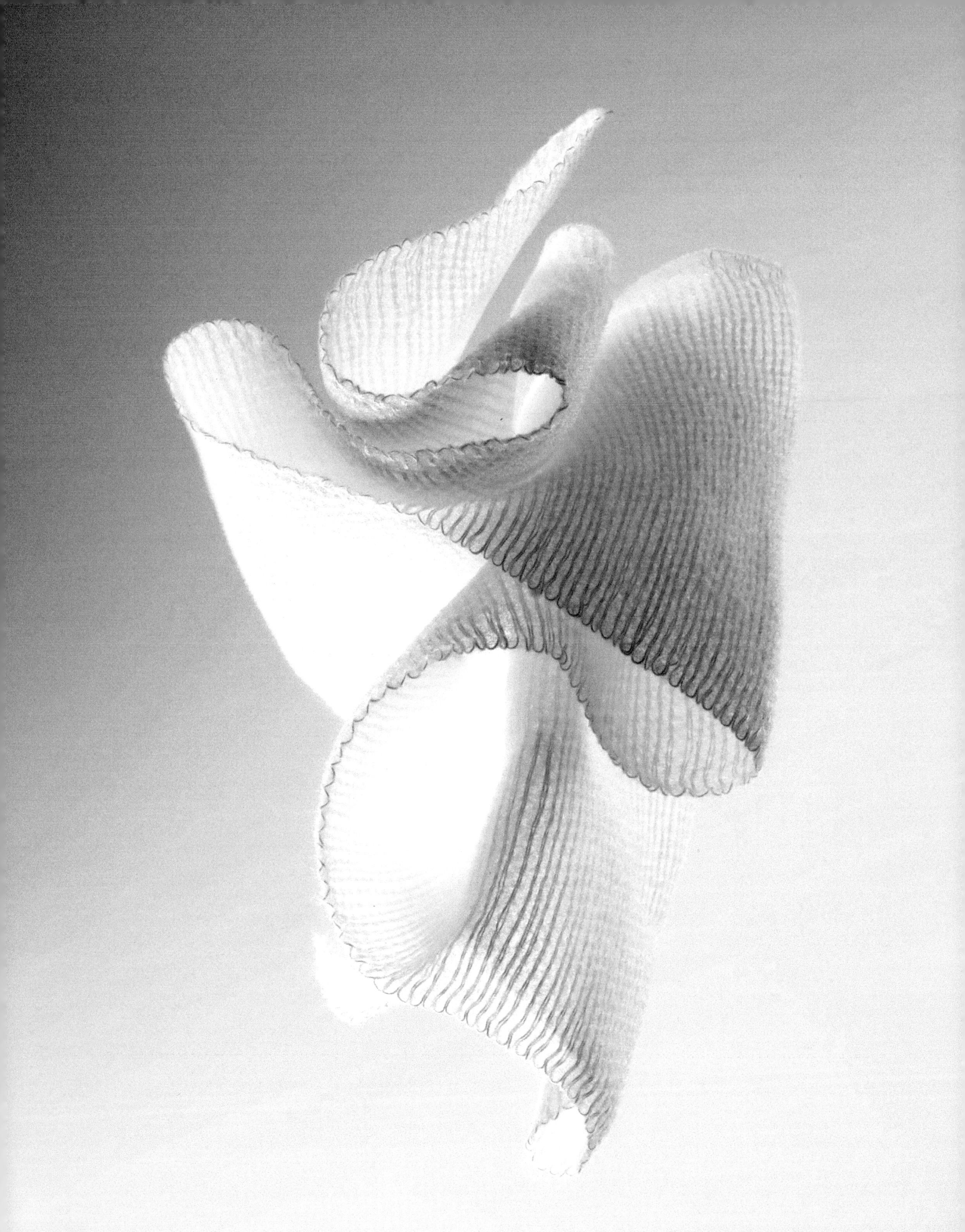

about the co–authors and editors

Aarent Brand Kanters, MD

Completed medical training at Maastricht University and went on to conduct research in liposculpture treatments following breast reconstruction. His doctoral studies at UMC Utrecht focused on investigating the efficacy of blood thinners in atherosclerosis. Today, as a cosmetic doctor, he specializes in facial and body injectable treatments and minor surgery at UMA Clinic. He is also a key figure in training other cosmetic doctors at UMA Academy, and he conducts innovative research into new cosmetic techniques and protocols at UMA Research.

Tom Decates, MD PhD

Aesthetic Physician in Amsterdam, the Netherlands, with a PhD in the origin of adverse events after soft tissue filler injections. One of the first academics in the field of aesthetic medicine with numerous publications to his name. Very experienced clinician and expert in the treatment of soft tissue fillers complications.

Rebecca Fitzgerald, MD

Board–certified dermatologist at a private practice in Los Angeles, California, with aesthetic injectables including fillers and neuromodulators as area of expertise. Sought–after teacher and speaker on the national and international stage. Publicist of many peer reviewed articles and textbook chapters and member of multiple advisory boards of leading dermatology societies.

Prof. Dr. Benoit Hendrickx, MD PhD

Associate professor in plastic surgery at the Brussels University Hospital (Belgium). Owner of several private practices. Sought–after trainer of facial anatomy and treatments using muscle relaxants and fillers. Keynote speaker at international conferences on facial anatomy and technology. Member of many international plastic surgery societies.

about the co–authors and editors

Jonathan Kadouch, MD PhD
Dermatologist, PhD in permanent filler complications and lecturer about the prevention and management of soft tissue filler complications. Author of a growing number of publications and contributor to the UMA Academy book publication on soft tissue filler complication prevention and management.

Prof. Peerooz Saeed, MD PhD
Global leader and educator in oculoplastic and orbit surgery, Peerooz is professor at the Amsterdam University Medical Center and offers aesthetic periorbital surgery at UMA Clinic. Among his extensive list of publications, he has contributed greatly in the algorithms published for management of acute visual loss afters soft tissue filler complications.

Leonie Schelke, MD PhD
Dutch certified aesthetic physician, with a private practice in Amsterdam for 20 years. Active at the policlinic for filler complications of the Department of Dermatology at Erasmus MC (Rotterdam the Netherlands). PhD in the use of duplex ultrasound and the management of filler complications. Co–founder and trainer at an organization for ultrasound courses in aesthetic medicine and dermatology.

Pieter Siebenga, MD PhD
Aesthetic Physician, leading the UMA Research department with profound knowledge of scientific research. Talented clinician, and a rising star in aesthetic training and education. Enthusiast of the scientific and clinical approach to male aesthetics and male attractiveness.

Job Thuis, MD
Aesthetic Physician, Chef de Clinique of UMA Clinic Global key–opinion leader, international lecturer and contributor to various research projects in aesthetic medicine. Very experienced in HA, Radiesse™ and botulinum toxin combination treatments. Expert status in more invasive procedures body contouring treatments as well.

Fred T.M. Tjan, MD
Dutch certified aesthetic physician owner of a private practice in The Hague, the Netherlands for over 20 years. Very active and known expert in the areas of biostimulatory injectables and soft tissue fillers.

Peter Velthuis, MD PhD
Dermatologist, practicing cosmetic dermatology since 1993. PhD in the area of photoimmunobiology. Over 20 years experience in his own private practice. Experienced in lasers applications, ultrasound imaging, injectables, liposuction and hair transplants. Academic at Erasmus Medical Center (Rotterdam, The Netherlands), chairing the cosmetic dermatology unit of the Department of Dermatology.

Ruscha Wijdeveld
Research assistant at UMA Research and member of the development team for learning materials at UMA Academy. Aesthetic medicine enthusiast and aspiring aesthetic physician.

Jani van Loghem, MD PhD

All our stories begin long before we were born. Jani van Loghem's starts with his grandparents. As pioneering immunologists, the pair travelled the world establishing a nascent medical field, training fellow doctors and changing lives. Their legacy also inspired a young Jani to complete medical school - where he naturally vowed to stay out of the unethical world of commercial medicine.

It was while working as a junior doctor in the general surgery department, that he first encountered the world of injectables - and it was love at first sight. The positivity one brought to patients' lives. The lack of superiors to boss one around. Jani began diving into the literature, taking workshops and going to aesthetic conferences. And the more he learned, the more he realised he needed to learn. Just like his grandparents before him, Jani was at the forefront of a new medical speciality. Merely running a successful clinic was not enough – he had the chance to be part of its development.

Jani's relentless passion for aesthetic medicine was key to the Netherlands being the first country in the world to recognise it as a two year specialism. Since then, his work has taken him around the world, sharing his experience and understanding with other professionals so that everyone can raise their game.

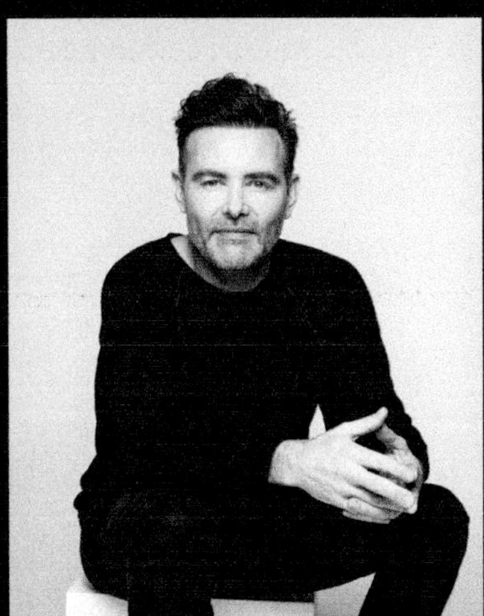

Philippe Snozzi, MD

Driving Philippe Snozzi is his great desire to change aesthetic medicine for the better. After graduating in medicine from the University of Zurich, Philippe practiced internal medicine and neurology, with a particular interest in the treatment of migraine patients with botulinum toxin, starting an extensive professional journey in the field of non-surgical aesthetic medicine. Fast–forward to today, and Philippe is globally respected aesthetic physicians and a renowned international expert in injectables.

Philippe first came across aesthetic medicine while working in internal medicine, substituting for an absent doctor friend. It surprised him how little was evidence–based unlike his own medical specialities. Yet he really liked its combination of social sciences and the chance to make a positive change in people's lives. He wrote, then shelved, his first clinic business plan around 2005, and it took bumping into his future business partner randomly three times in various locations, including a club in LA, before realizing the universe was telling him to take his plan seriously. In 2007 they set up one of the leading Swiss clinics in Zurich and ran it successfully ever since.

Now Philippe has authored and co–authored multiple publications, and lectures nationally and internationally with a special interest in teaching prevention and management of filler complications. He loves sharing his learnings—and what still needs to be learned—with other professionals.

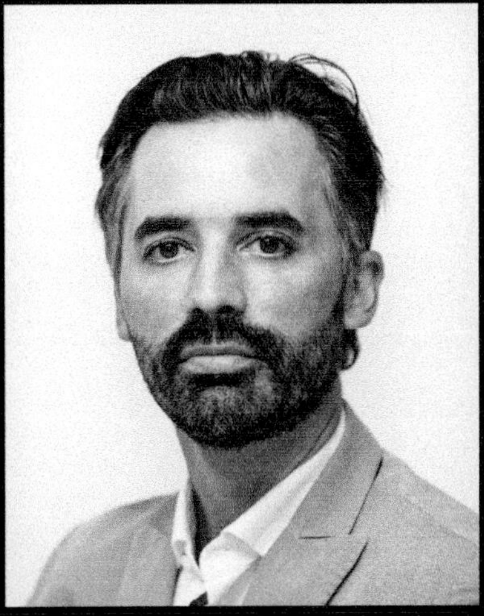

This book unveils his insights and is set to improve practitioners' knowledge based on empirical evidence. What advice would Philippe give his former self? "Don't worry too much about things in life. Even worst case scenarios tend to turn out much better than anticipated."

our curriculum

Our curriculum of book publications, webinars, discourses and hands-on training is created by the same team who developed The Netherlands' medical specialty of aesthetic medicine. Tailor-made for the digital age, our courses combine a solid theoretical background with clinical training, with unprecedented access to the expertise of some of the industry's top practitioners.

toxins

toxin essentials

advanced toxin techniques

soft tissue fillers

filler essentials

advanced filler techniques

complication prevention & management

attractiveness

female beauty

male attractiveness

intimate areas

aesthetic surgery

facial surgery

body contouring

oculoplastics

aesthetic skin therapy

energy based devices

chemical peels

needling and skin boosters

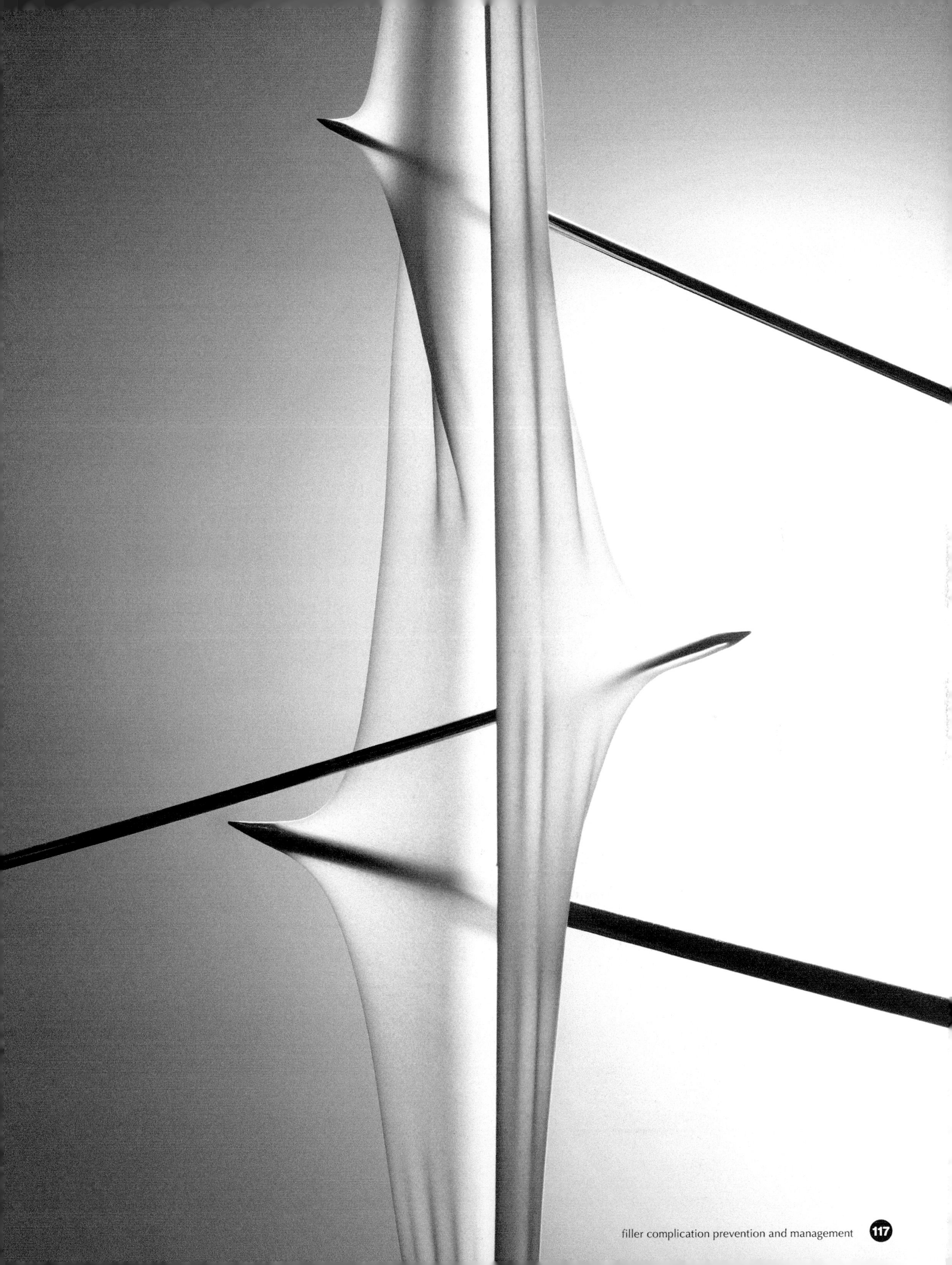

Index

A

Abscesses, 39, 86
Acne scars, 95
Allergan, 22
Allergens, 14
Angiosomes, 18, 47
Antibiotic treatment, for infection, 8, 39, 45, 50, 57, 75
Anticoagulants, 14, 31, 53
Aquamid, 74
Arterial anatomy, 13, 17
Arterial blockage, 85
Arterial occlusion, 47, 48, 86
Artery 3D, 100
Aspiration, 13, 22
Augmented Reality, 100

B

Belotero Balance, 33
Bio-alcamid, 74
Blindness, as complication of STF. *See* complications, STF
Blood thinners, 31
Bruising, 14, 31. *See also* complications, STF

C

Calcium hydroxylapatite (CaHA), 16, 29, 83
 CaHA-induced discoloration, 34
 CaHA-induced nodules, 42
 CaHA-induced retinal ischemia, 57–58
Cannulas, 13, 14, 17, 20, 21, 22, 31, 38, 39
Cardiovascular risk profile, 31
Choke vessels, 18, 47, 56
Cohesive polydensified matrix (CPM), 33
Collagen, 42, 43, 58, 69, 74, 83, 94
Complications, STF
 blindness, 17, 46, 47, 85
 edema (*see* edema)
 infection (*see* infection, following STF)
 late inflammatory response syndrome (LIRS), 37, 42–45
 nodules (*see* nodules)
 patient history, risk associated with, 12, 14
 practitioner-related, 14, 17, 20, 21, 22, 48
 product type risks, 12, 16
 retinal ischemia, 53, 57–58
 skin discoloration (*see* skin discoloration)
 techniques, safest, 13
 vascular, 13, 18, 46–48, 49–50, 56–57
Corticosteroids, 36, 37, 45, 53, 96
COVID-19 vaccinations, 45
Cytokines, 32, 36, 43, 58, 71

D

Damage-associated molecular patterns (DAMPs), 71
Delayed onset nodules (DON). *See* late inflammatory response syndrome (LIRS)
DNA filler tests, 101
Doppler ultrasound (DUS) scans prior to STF. *See* ultrasound

E

Edema, 16
 hypersensitivity reactions, 36–37
 LIRS, as symptom of, 37, 44
 malar, 37
 overview, 35
 treatment, 37
Embolization, 17
Erbium-Yag laser, 37

F

Fibroblasts, 43, 58, 69, 71
Fibrosis, 31
Fitzpatrick skin types, 32, 61

G

Granulomas, 41, 43
 classifications, 69
 formation, 68
 GFBR, excessive, 72, 75
 grading, 69
 overview, 68
 pathology, 69, 71
 phagocytosis, 68
 symptoms, 71
Gunshot technique, 48

H

HA embolus, 50
Herpes simplex, 40
HoloLens2, 100
Human Leucocyte Antigen (HLA) complex, 14
Hyaluronic acid (HA), 16, 18, 29, 68, 72, 83, 86
Hyaluronidase (HYAL), 33, 44, 53, 93
Hyperpigmentation, 14, 30, 31, 32, 75
Hypertrophic scars, 95, 96
Hypoperfusion, 47
Hypoxemia, 18

I

Infection, following STF
 acute bacterial, 39
 fungemia, 38
 MRSA, 38
 necrotizing fascitis, 38
 overview, 38
 viral, 40
Inflammatory reactions, 16
Infrared facial heating, 100
Injection techniques, 14, 20, 21, 48
Interferon-gamma, 71
Intralesional laser therapy (ILT), 75
Ischemia, 30

J

Juvederm, 22, 33

K

Keloid scars, 95

L

Lanluma, 58, 59
Laser therapy, for complication management, 97, 99
Late inflammatory response syndrome (LIRS), 37, 42–45
Lidocaine, 93

M

Magnetic resonance angiography (MRA), 100
Methotrexate, 45
Minocycline, 75
MRSA, 38

N

Necrosis, 17, 49, 72
Needles, types of, 22, 48, 75
Neovascularization, 32
Nodules
 causes, 41
 delayed onset nodules (DON), 44
 early onset, inflammatory, 43
 early onset, non-inflammatory, 42
 late onset, inflammatory, 43–45
 late onset, non-inflammatory, 43
 late PLLA, 61
 non-inflammatory PLLA, 60
 overview, 41
 treatment, 45
Non-resorbable fillers, 73, 74, 75–76

O

Orbicularis retaining ligament (ORL), 37

P

Panniculitis, 86
Patient history, 12, 14
Pattern recognition receptors (PRR), 71
Peripheral ischemia, 50
Phagocytosis, 68
Poly methyl methacrylic acid (PMMA), 83
Poly-L-lactic acid (PLLA), 29, 48, 58, 59, 60, 61
Polyacrylamide hydrogel, 74
Polyalkylimide gel, 74
Post-treatment scarring, 94, 95, 96

Postinflammatory hyperpigmentation (PIH). *see* hyperpigmentation
Products, STF
risks associated with (*see* complications, STF)
storage, 93
types, 12, 16, 18, 22, 33
Puffiness, 16

R

Resilient HA (RHA), 33
Retinal artery, 46, 55
Retinal ischemia, 53
Retrobulbar injection, 55

S

S. pyogenes, 38
Safety and infection-prevention protocols, 39
Scar formation, 94, 95
Scars, types of, 95
Sculptra, 29, 48, 58, 59
Silicone, 74
Skin discoloration
ecchymosis, 31
hematoma, 30
hyperpigmentation (*see* hyperpigmentation)
neovascularization, 32
overview, 30
Tyndall effect, 30, 33
yellowish, 34
Soft tissue filler (STF) injections
complications (*see* complications, STF)
non-resorbable (*see* non-resorbable fillers)
permanent, 74
product types, 12

T

Tattoo removal, with lasers, 99
Time of Flight, 100
Toll-like receptors, 71
Tumor necrosis factor (TNF), 71
Tyndall effect, 30, 33

U

Ultra, 22
Ultrasound
device, overview of, 86
doppler ultrasound (DUS) scans prior to STF, 47–48
filler complications, used in, 86
filler images, 83
overview, 82
pre-treatment assessment, 85
ultrasound-guided injections, 86
UMA fuller first aid kit, 92
Uticaria, 36

V

Vaccinations and LIRS, 45
Valaciclovir, 40
Vascular adverse effect (VAE), 85
Vascular compromise, 46, 47
Vascular obstructions, 50
Vascular occlusion, 18
Vitamin K cream, 31
Vycross, 33

Z

Zygomatico-cutaneous ligament (ZCL), 37